THE PRINCIPLES OF MENTAL CARE

*A Systems Approach
to Building Resilience in Children*

SATORU ISAKA, PH.D.

The Principles of Mental Care

Disclaimer:

This book is not intended as a substitute for medical advice. The reader should regularly consult a physician in matters relating to health, and particularly with respect to any symptoms that may require diagnosis or medical attention. The exercises and advice in this book are given for informational purposes only. Consult a physician before performing this or any health regimen.

The content of this book is for general instruction only. Each person's physical, emotional, and spiritual condition is unique. The instruction in this book is not intended to replace or interrupt the reader's relationship with a physician or other professional. Please consult your doctor for matters pertaining to your specific health and diet.

To contact the author, visit www.visiondelmar.com.

ISBN: 978-1721938025

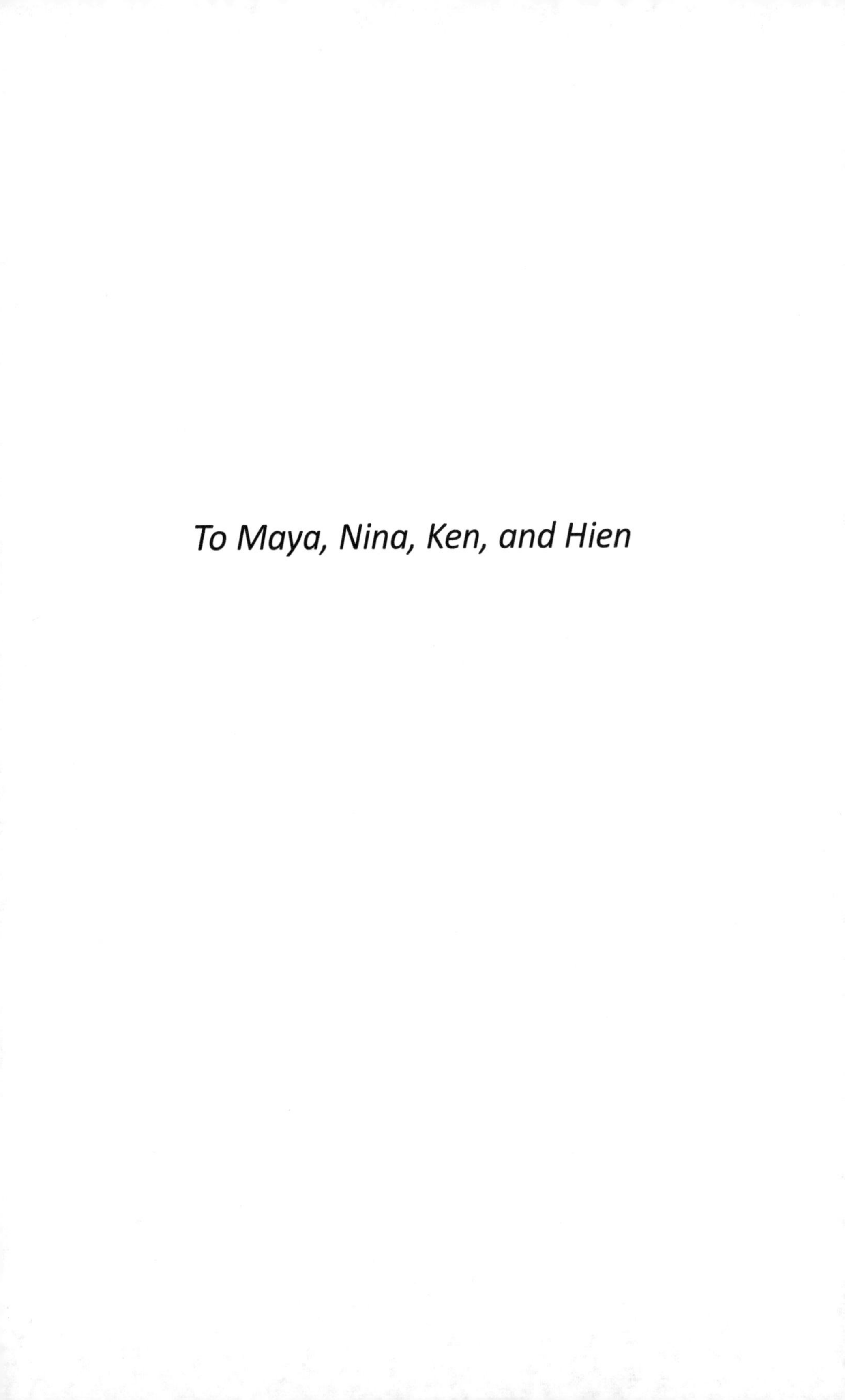

To Maya, Nina, Ken, and Hien

CONTENTS

PROLOGUE

LIFE MAY SEEM fine when things are going well, but it can change at any moment. All of a sudden, the world becomes a lonely place. Feelings are invisible, but they are the most important factor in our well-being. As recent studies show,[1] the current treatment options for mental health are limited and inadequate. It's time to rethink mental health, and find a systematic approach to prevention, especially for young children to build resilience. Because everyone has good days and bad days, every child and adult should know how to perform routine mental care, just like dental care. What is mental care? That's what this book is about. This book establishes the principles of mental care from a systems science perspective to promote a practical, systematic approach to mental wellness.

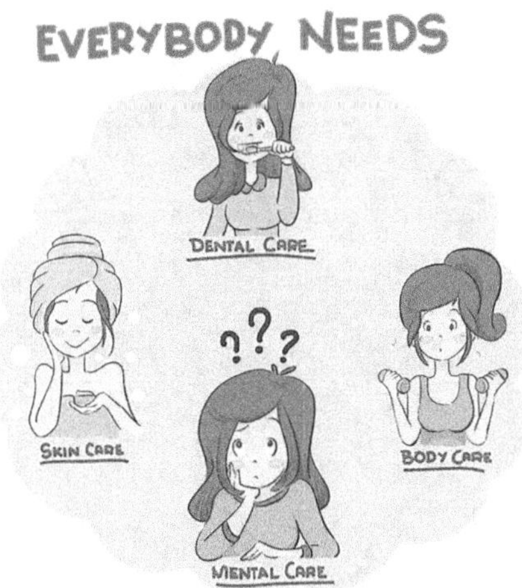

1. For example, Cox GR, Callahan P, Churchill R, Hunot V, Merry SN, Parker AG, Hetrick SE. Psychological therapies versus antidepressant medication, alone and in combination for depression in children and adolescents. Cochrane Database of Systematic Reviews 2014, Issue 11. Art. No.: CD008324.

HOW TO USE THIS BOOK

I WROTE THIS BOOK primarily for parents and caregivers with young children. This is not a book of psychology, brain science, or how to raise children. There are plenty of books for that in bookstores and libraries. This book is about systems and principles of mental care.

Imagine building and sending a rocket to the Moon without understanding the underlying principles of science. It would be difficult and frustrating, wouldn't it? Well, human brains are far more complex and unknown than rockets. The world we live is more crowded and chaotic than the Moon. Now we are sending our children into an environment where people increasingly rely on medications and therapies to maintain their main control unit, the brain. Think about that for a minute.

I did think about that when I was raising my three children. My conclusion was that I needed to build resilience in children. I think many of you would agree. No matter how young or small they may be, children are each unique individuals with their own feelings and thinking in their environment. It would be foolish to think that we could control and protect them throughout their lives. But, like giving them vaccines to strengthen their immune systems, we could help them enhance their skills and knowledge of mental health, so that when they grow up, they could figure out their own ways of preserving their mental, physical, and social well-being.

I researched and came across a lot of philosophical conjectures with anecdotal evidence in psychology, mental health, and parenting. They were inspiring, but when it comes to pragmatic matters in mental health care, lack of principles was evident. How do healthcare systems treat mental health and why? How do psychiatric medications and therapies work and why? How do education systems teach mental health and why? Is there an equivalent to dental care in mental care according to public health policies?

Answers to these questions are surprisingly unclear, and we have to dig deep to get a good handle on these important topics. My hope is that this book brings clarity and structure to mental health, and offers a positive, constructive outlook with practical resources for parents and caregivers to use to build resilience in children.

I know how busy my target readers are as they raise children while maintaining a healthy work-life balance. It shouldn't be difficult to read this book from beginning to the end, but you don't need to. Feel free to skip any section you find not useful, but please don't just read and do nothing. Please take a few of the preventive actions described in the book.

The book is divided into three parts: analysis, synthesis, and resource. Each part has three chapters. The first part reviews and analyzes how mental health is currently handled in the health-care system and identifies what the problems are. The second part provides solutions to the problems. The last part provides practical resources for mental care.

My writing style may reflect critical views toward health care as an industry. I have great respect and appreciation for people in health care, but the cold fact is that prevention is not their main business. I hope this book motivates readers to rethink mental health by thinking of science and prevention, especially with children in mind.

Notes on Terminology

I CHOSE TO USE the phrase "mental care" as opposed to "mental health care" for a reason.

In this book, the words health and wellness are distinguished in the following sense: health is about medical condition; wellness is about life quality. Even though the World Health Organization (WHO) defines health as a state of complete physical, mental, and social well-being, the reality is that health is treated as a medical condition of illness and injury by healthcare providers, insurers, and policymakers.

Wellness, on the other hand, is a generally accepted term that implies the quality of general well-being. The word wellness is actually better aligned with WHO's definition of health than the word health itself in practice. To signify its focus on wellness for the purpose of prevention and preservation, the phrase "mental care" is used in this book. The phrase "mental health care" is only used in context related to health care and the healthcare industry.

PART 1

ANALYSIS

THE FIRST SECTION of this book is about fact-finding in current mental healthcare. Chapter 1 identifies the underlying problems in mental health. Chapter 2 analyzes the first treatment option in mental health care — psychiatric medications. Chapter 3 analyzes the second treatment option in mental health care — psychotherapies.

CHAPTER 1

THE CURRENT STATE OF MENTAL HEALTH

1.1. The problems

A man was stressed at work. He feared he might lose his job. He had no history of mental health problems, but lately he felt anxious and couldn't sleep well. One day, he decided to ask his primary care doctor for help. The doctor prescribed a medication for anxiety and another medication for insomnia. The drugs didn't help. He returned to see the doctor three times in a few weeks. At each visit, the medication dose was increased. Two weeks after the last doctor visit, the man shot and killed himself.

MEDICATION IS CURRENTLY the first choice in the treatment of mental illness. A government study[2] shows that one in ten Americans takes antidepressant medication. Antidepressants are the third most commonly prescribed drug for Americans of all ages. That's a concern, but the most disturbing statistic is that 80 percent of those antidepressants were prescribed by non-psychiatrists without any accompanying psychiatric diagnosis.[3]

If the medications actually worked, such statistics might not be a big issue. Unfortunately, the efficacy of current psychiatric treatment is questionable. In November 2014, an independent research organization, Cochrane, published a concerning report on the **efficacy of medication and psychotherapies** for treating depression in children and adolescents[4]. The report concluded: *"On the basis of the available evidence, we do not know whether psychological therapy, antidepressant medication or a combination of the two is most effective to treat depressive disorders in children and adolescents."*

In June 2015, T. R. Insel, then the director of the National Institute of Mental Health, issued a stern warning: *"four decades of drug development resulting in over 20 antipsychotics and over 30 antidepressants have not demonstrably reduced the morbidity or mortality of mental disorders."*[5] Simply put, medications and therapies — the current treatment options for mental health — are limited in their effectiveness and inadequate.

To make matters worse, the quality of psychology research in general also has been found to be questionable. According to an analysis by Open Science Collaboration published in August 2015, two-thirds of published psychology experiments failed reproducibility tests[6]. In other words, scientific claims made by these psychology studies may not be reliable. Because all psychotherapies are based on psychology research studies, this is a concerning discovery.

In the meantime, there is a crisis going on at the front line of clinical care — the emergency room. The National Association of State Mental Health Program Directors reported a survey of more than 6,000 emergency departments nationwide. Seventy percent reported boarding psychiatric patients for hours or days, and 10 percent boarded patients for several weeks.[7] The American College of Emergency Physicians points out the problem: *"Limited funding, limited resources, and patient placement difficulties have accumulated to the current crisis of mental health patients boarding in the emergency department."*[8]

Today, one in five American adults experiences a mental health issue in a year, and one in five youths aged 13 to 18 experiences a severe mental disorder at some point during his or her life.[15] The global cost of mental health care is projected to exceed $6 trillion in 2030 — larger than the cost of cancer, diabetes, and chronic respiratory diseases combined.[16] What can we do?

Prevention

It is easy to understand why healthcare is having difficulty dealing with mental health. First of all, neuroscientists are still trying to figure out how our brains work. Unlike physical illness such as flu or pneumonia, mental states are invisible and difficult to measure objectively. There is nothing like a thermometer or blood sampling to test for mental illness. Diagnosis and treatment relies only on what and how patients complain about their feelings and conditions, or on behavior observed by someone else. This subjective and qualitative nature of mental health data makes it difficult to design a reproducible solution.

Variability in root causes also poses challenges. Everyone is different. Everyone has different values, faces different obstacles in life, and is immersed in different environments. And most importantly, everyone feels and reacts differently to stressors. This is because everyone has a different genetic makeup, neural development and adaptation, biochemical balance, environmental exposure and circumstances, and in some cases, underlying biological disorder. This variability within populations poses major obstacles for scientific studies to generate reproducible outcomes and to come up with guidelines for public health and clinical practice. These reasons may explain why most people don't know what to do with mental health.

The answer may reside in considering what we have done in the past when treatment for a certain illness is difficult. We opt for preventive care. Think about flu, for example. Flu is caused by a virus and there is no cure for viral infection.[18] So we take preventive measures seriously. First, we educate ourselves to minimize the chance of being infected by virus, like washing hands for example. Second, we build resilience. In the case of flu, we strengthen our immune systems by taking a vaccination when available.

These are helpful, but the most effective way to build resilience is to strengthen our daily lifestyle and build up our overall well-being. Good habits of hydration, nutrition, exercise, and sleep go a long way toward building resilience against illness in general. We teach our children these types of skills and knowledge, starting at a young age. Therefore, the best course of action for mental health is building resilience for prevention and preservation. The question is how?

1.2. Academic work on mental health

The World Health Organization (WHO) released a report in 2004 promoting the concept of evidence-based prevention and promotion in mental health.[9] In 2009, the Institute of Medicine (now the National Academy of Medicine) published a report also presenting the idea of preventive mental health for young people.[10] In 2010, WHO released a comprehensive action plan for mental health.[11] Some researchers, for example[12], propose a broad approach to mental health by promoting both positive well-being and prevention.

These grand visions are rooted in a population-based public health model. According to the Surgeon General's report on mental health, a public health approach "encompasses a focus on epidemiological surveillance, health promotion, disease prevention, and access to service."[13] Epidemiological surveillance means systematically collecting and analyzing health data for public health programs. In other words, a public health approach is a big task of collecting a massive amount of data from broad target populations, and then thoroughly analyzing them before a solution can be derived. Considering the breadth of topics to be negotiated, including education, economics, government policies, social service, parenting, and partnerships with health-care systems, the public health approach is overwhelmingly ambitious and long-term in its return on investment. For that reason, some researchers, for example[14], argue that we need to combine public health models with clinical practice for patients with early signs of disorder within primary care.

How does prevention work? According to WHO[9], "preventive interventions work by focusing on reducing risk factors and enhancing protective factors associated with mental ill-health."

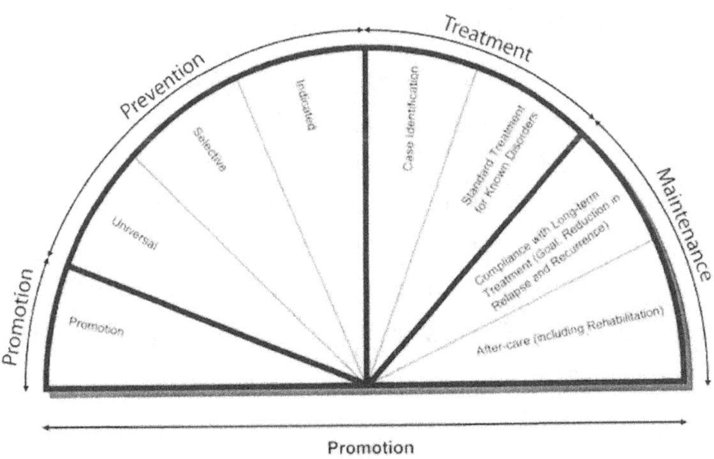

Figure 1. Mental health intervention spectrum (Institute of Medicine 2009)

Unfortunately, the academic work on preventive interventions do not offer practical solutions. Currently there is no standard structure to capture and represent risk and protective factors. There is no quantitative measurement tool. Time-consuming psychiatric evaluations are the only way to identify specific risk factors for individuals today, and such evaluation only takes place when the patient is already suffering from severe symptoms.

1.3. Clinical practice on mental health

As mental health comes to the forefront of preventive care strategies for patients, the **primary care providers** (PCP), like family practitioners and pediatricians, find that more attention needs to be paid to patients' mental wellness during primary care office visits. This is because the highest impact on care quality, resource use, and patient satisfaction comes at the initial assessment and treatment stage, as shown in Figure 2. When you have a medical issue, PCPs are the doctors you would contact first, as most health insurance policies require.

Unfortunately, when it comes to mental health issues, no thorough psychiatric assessment is possible by PCPs for two reasons. First, there is not enough time available in the current primary care setting. It could take several hours to complete a psychiatric assessment, but PCPs normally can only afford about 15 minutes per patient at a time. Second, performing a psychiatric assessment requires special skill training and clinical experience. PCPs are not trained in this area. These skills and experience belong to psychiatrists and clinical psychologists.

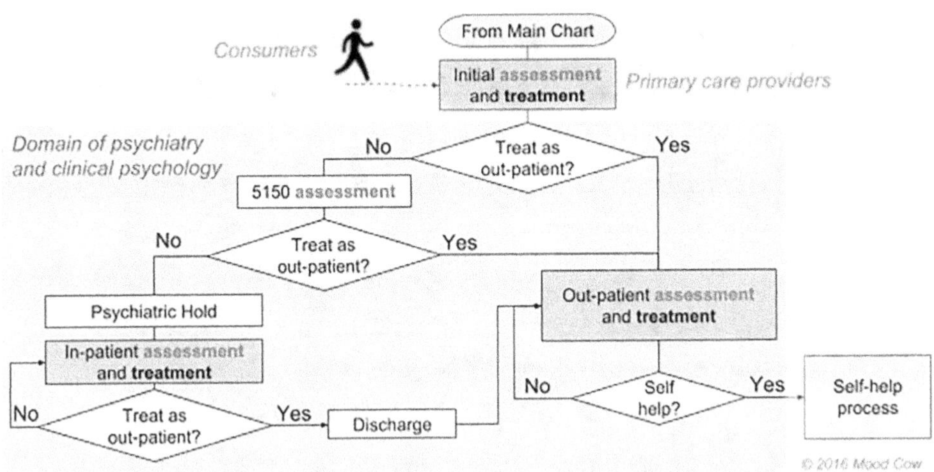

Figure 2. Health-care provider process

At the initial assessment stage, PCPs now use abbreviated screening questionnaires called PHQ-9 for depression and GAD-7 for anxiety to evaluate the presence and severity of mental health disorders. PHQ-9 and GAD-7 were developed by Drs. R.L. Spitzer, J.B.W. Williams, and K. Kroenke in the 1990s with financial support from the pharmaceutical giant, Pfizer Inc.[17] The objective was to offer clinical tools that would enable primary care physicians to quickly identify mental health disorders and arrive at clinical reasons to prescribe medications for them. The questionnaires are short; 9 questions in PHQ-9 (Figure 3), 7 in GAD-7 (Figure 4). The nature of the questions is apparently designed to minimize false-negatives to avoid missing the opportunity to catch early signs of mental disorder. However, this regimen ends up increasing the occurrence of false-positives, which is not necessarily a problem as long as the tests are used properly.

PHQ-9 and GAD-7 are early screeners and quick-assessment tools, not diagnostic tools. Unfortunately, the screeners have been used as a diagnostic tool by PCPs. As a result, they became the catalyst for the increased use of psychiatric medications in recent years. The issue is not the tools; it's the process in health care.

PATIENT HEALTH QUESTIONNAIRE-9
(PHQ-9)

Over the <u>last 2 weeks</u>, how often have you been bothered by any of the following problems? *(Use "✔" to indicate your answer)*	Not at all	Several days	More than half the days	Nearly every day
1. Little interest or pleasure in doing things	0	1	2	3
2. Feeling down, depressed, or hopeless	0	1	2	3
3. Trouble falling or staying asleep, or sleeping too much	0	1	2	3
4. Feeling tired or having little energy	0	1	2	3
5. Poor appetite or overeating	0	1	2	3
6. Feeling bad about yourself — or that you are a failure or have let yourself or your family down	0	1	2	3
7. Trouble concentrating on things, such as reading the newspaper or watching television	0	1	2	3
8. Moving or speaking so slowly that other people could have noticed? Or the opposite — being so fidgety or restless that you have been moving around a lot more than usual	0	1	2	3
9. Thoughts that you would be better off dead or of hurting yourself in some way	0	1	2	3

FOR OFFICE CODING   _0_   + _______ + _______ + _______

=Total Score: _______

Figure 3. Patient Health Questionnaire (PHQ-9)

GAD-7				
Over the <u>last 2 weeks</u>, how often have you been bothered by the following problems? *(Use "✔" to indicate your answer)*	Not at all	Several days	More than half the days	Nearly every day
1. Feeling nervous, anxious or on edge	0	1	2	3
2. Not being able to stop or control worrying	0	1	2	3
3. Worrying too much about different things	0	1	2	3
4. Trouble relaxing	0	1	2	3
5. Being so restless that it is hard to sit still	0	1	2	3
6. Becoming easily annoyed or irritable	0	1	2	3
7. Feeling afraid as if something awful might happen	0	1	2	3

(For office coding: Total Score T____ = ____ + ____ + ____)

Figure 4. Generalized Anxiety Disorder Questionnaire (GAD-7)

While PHQ-9 and GAD-7 are quick screening tools, there exists a comprehensive diagnostic manual for psychiatric evaluation. The Diagnostic and Statistical Manual of Mental Disorders (DSM) published by the American Psychiatric Association is the universal authority in the US for psychiatric diagnosis, treatment recommendations, and insurance payment criteria. It is important to recognize that DSM is definitive in the sense of its standardized use in this country, not in the sense of its scientific accuracy and reliability. The psychiatric diagnostic categories are still subjective and symptom-based.

DSM is also an important resource for general public to understand how psychiatric illnesses are defined, and how clinicians and insurance companies diagnose and treat patients. Because diagnostic categories are symptom-based, how you present your symptoms to clinicians affect decisions on treatment and insurance coverage.

A case in point is autism. In 2013, when DSM was revised from its previous edition, significant changes to the criteria and categories of autism took place. The previously separated diagnostic labels of Autistic Disorder, Asperger's Disorder, and Pervasive Developmental Disorder Not Otherwise Specified (PDD-NOS) were replaced by a single umbrella term called "Autistic Spectrum Disorder (ASD)" with severity levels. Unfortunately, this change affected millions of people who were already receiving treatment and insurance coverage based on their previous diagnoses. The reason for this label change was not scientific. There was no new scientific discovery or new diagnostic or treatment methods that motivated the change in categorization. It was merely for procedural improvement that benefits clinicians and insurance companies. Interested readers are encouraged to read further on autism and DSM.

The Autism Research Institute on DSM-5 https://www.autism. com/news_dsmV

The American Psychiatric Association on DSM-5 https://www. psychiatry.org/psychiatrists/practice/dsm

The Center for Disease Control and Prevention on DSM-5 https://www.cdc.gov/ncbddd/autism/hcp-dsm.html

1.4. Systems view on mental health maintenance

Our mind is not completely observable from the outside, and everyone reacts differently to stressful events or situations. Mental states are invisible, not well-defined, and not consistently diagnosable. Therefore, an attempt from outside to regulate an unobservable system is prone to make the system unstable. According to this systems science principle, applying external treatment such as medications based solely on symptom complaints carries a risk of negative impact on system stability.

Unfortunately, that's how the current mental health care system is structured to act, as shown in Figure 5. The screening tests such as PHQ-9 and GAD-7 assess symptoms only, without reflecting possible causes and stressors. In the current primary-care setting, the protocol allows for a quick assessment of symptoms that directly results in a clinical decision to medicate the patient.

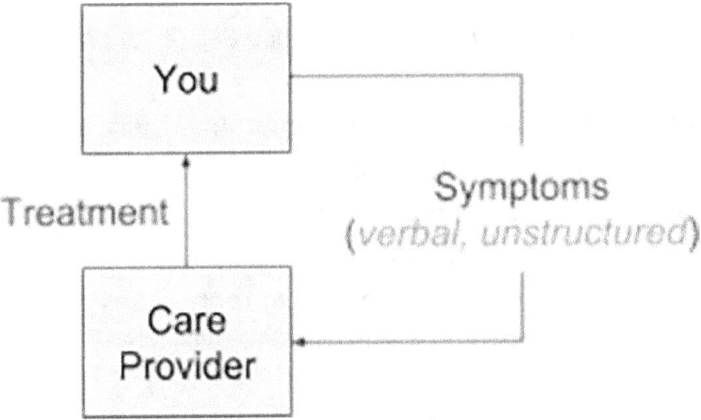

Figure 5. Current mental care system

Let us step back and take a look at mental health as a maintenance process. There are two types of maintenance: preventive and corrective.

Preventive maintenance is a process of taking actions to eliminate or minimize future corrective actions. Changing the oil in your car or brushing your teeth are examples of preventive maintenance.

Corrective maintenance is a process of taking actions to repair functional failure. Replacing engine parts or filling a tooth cavity is an example of corrective maintenance.

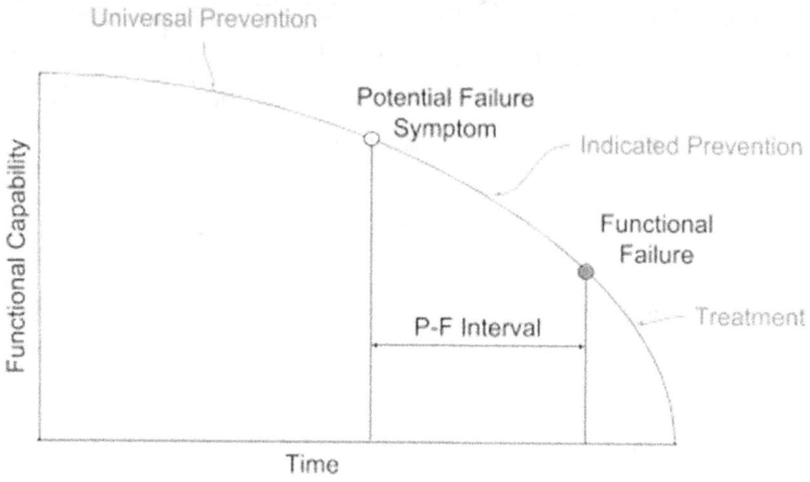

Figure 6. P-F curve and mental health intervention

Prevention is not all about treating symptoms. There are two objectives in prevention. First, universal prevention. The goal of **universal prevention** is to identify potential root causes and take actions to reduce their effect. Contaminated lubricant in your engine or sugar in your mouth are examples of root causes of potential failure in the future. That's why you periodically change oil or brush teeth.

Once you see smoke coming from your car or you feel pain in your tooth, it becomes a matter of time before the problem gets worse. In engineering, this is called a P-F interval (Figure 6), the amount of time that elapses between the detection of a potential failure and its deterioration to functional failure. This is where the second objective of prevention — indicated prevention — comes in. The goal of **indicated prevention** is to maximize the P-F interval to avoid functional failure as long as possible.

Here's how this works in the health-care system today: When a symptom affects your life quality, you reach out to a health-care provider to receive appropriate **treatment** to address the symptoms. The current health-care system treats psychiatric medications as a means to correct the problems; however, these medications are originally designed to suppress the symptoms, not correct the root cause. Because of this, addressing symptom complaints by using psychiatric medications cannot be considered as corrective action, just as taking a painkiller will not treat tooth decay. Perhaps it is more appropriate to think of medications as an indicated prevention tool that prolongs the P-F interval, rather than as a corrective tool. This distinction and understanding of the role of medications in mental health is important.

In the following chapters, we analyze medications and therapies for mental health.

References

2. Pratt LA, Brody DJ, Gu Q. Antidepressant use in persons aged 12 and over: United States, 2005–2008. *NCHS Data Brief*. National Center for Health Statistics. 2011. https://www.ncbi.nlm.nih.gov/pubmed/22617183

3. Mojtabai R. Olfson M. Proportion Of Antidepressants Prescribed Without A Psychiatric Diagnosis Is Growing. *Health Affairs*. 2011;30(8):1434-1442. https://www.ncbi.nlm.nih.gov/pubmed/21821561

4. Cox GR, Callahan P, Churchill R, Hunot V, Merry SN, Parker AG, Hetrick SE. Psychological therapies versus antidepressant medication, alone and in combination for depression in children and adolescents. *Cochrane Database of Systematic Reviews* 2014, Issue 11. Art. No.: CD008324. https://www.ncbi.nlm.nih.gov/pubmed/23152255

5. Insel TR. The NIMH experimental medicine initiative. *World Psychiatry*. 2015;14(2):151-153. https://www.ncbi.nlm.nih.gov/pmc/articles/PMC4471962/

6. Open Science Collaboration. Estimating the reproducibility of psychological science. *Science*, 349(6251), aac4716. 2015. https://www.ncbi.nlm.nih.gov/pubmed/26315443

7.   Glover RW. Miller JE, Sadowski SR. Proceedings on the state budget crisis and the behavioral health treatment gap: The impact on public substance abuse and mental health systems. NASMHPD. 2012. https://www.nasmhpd.org/sites/default/files/SummaryCongressional%20Briefing_2012(6).pdf

8.   American College of Emergency Physicians. Practical Solutions to Boarding of Psychiatric Patients in the Emergency Department. October 2015. http://www.macep.org/Files/Behavioral%20Health%20Boarding/Practical%20Solutions%20to%20Boarding%20of%20Psych%20Patients%20in%20EDs.pdf

9.   World Health Organization. Prevention of Mental Disorders: Effective Interventions and Policy Options. Geneva: World Health Organization, 2004. http://www.who.int/mental_health/evidence/en/prevention_of_mental_disorders_sr.pdf

10.   National Research Council (US) and Institute of Medicine (US) Committee on the Prevention of Mental Disorders and Substance Abuse Among Children, Youth, and Young Adults: Research Advances and Promising Interventions; O'Connell ME, Boat T, Warner KE, editors. Preventing Mental, Emotional, and Behavioral Disorders Among Young People: Progress and Possibilities. Washington (DC): National Academies Press (US); 2009. https://www.ncbi.nlm.nih.gov/books/NBK32775/

11.   World Health Organization. Comprehensive mental health action plan 2013-2020. Geneva: World Health Organization, 2004. http://www.who.int/mental_health/action_plan_2013/en/

12.   Wahlbeck K. Public mental health: the time is ripe for translation of evidence into practice. *World Psychiatry*. 2015;14(1):36-42. https://www.ncbi.nlm.nih.gov/pmc/articles/PMC4329888/

13.   US Department of Health and Human Services. Mental health: A report of the Surgeon General, Rockville,, MD. US Department of Health and Human Services, Substance Abuse and Mental Health Services Administration, Center

for Mental Health Services, National Institutes of Health, National Institute of Mental Health. 1999. https://profiles.nlm.nih.gov/ps/retrieve/ResourceMetadata/NNBBHS

14. Weissman MM. Applied public mental health: bridging the gap between evidence and clinical practice. *World Psychiatry*. 2015;14(1):45-47. https://www.ncbi.nlm.nih.gov/pmc/articles/PMC4329891/

15. Mental Health By the Numbers. National Alliance on Mental Illness. 2015. https://www.nami.org/Learn-More/Mental-Health-By-the-Numbers

16. Bloom DE. Cafiero ET. et al. The Global Economic Burden of Noncommunicable Diseases. Geneva: World Economic Forum. 2011. http://www3.weforum.org/docs/WEF_Harvard_HE_GlobalEconomicBurdenNonCommunicableDiseases_2011.pdf

17. Pfizer. Patient Health Questionnaire (PHQ) Screeners. Retrieved from http://www.phqscreeners.com/select-screener/

18. US National Library of Medicine. Virus Infection. MedlinePlus. Retrieved from https://medlineplus.gov/viralinfections.html

CHAPTER 2

MEDICATIONS AND SUPPLEMENTS

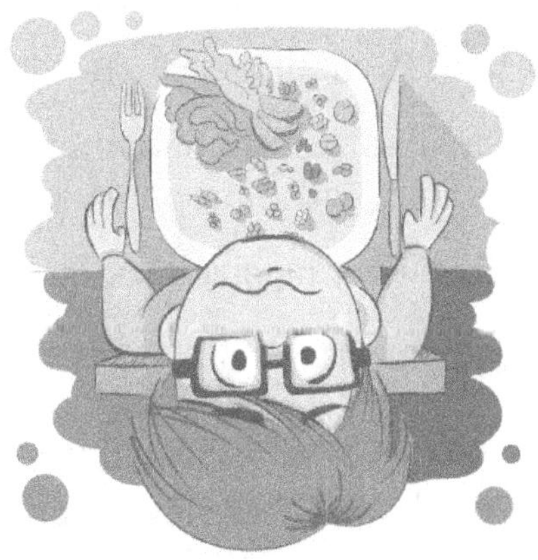

2.1. Psychiatric medications

Medications are chemical substances. A chemical substance that changes one's brain function is called a psychoactive drug.[19] The reason for using medications for mental health is to use psychoactive drugs to **biochemically control how you feel and think**. Because of the inherent risks associated with biochemical treatment, medications should only be administered for disabling problems that cannot be regulated by other means of treatment.

In practice, however, medications are far more commonly prescribed than is necessary. Remember: According to a government study, roughly **one in ten Americans takes antidepressants**[20] and they are the **third most commonly prescribed drug** for Americans (after cholesterol treatments and pain-killers). Disturbingly, **80% of antidepressants were prescribed by non-psychiatrists without any accompanying psychiatric diagnosis.**[21]

According to the National Institute of Mental Health (NIMH), five common types of psychiatric medications are used today.[22]

- **Antidepressants:** Treat depression, anxiety, pain, insomnia, ADHD.

- **Anti-anxiety medications:** Reduce symptoms of anxiety, panic attacks.

- **Stimulants:** Treat attention deficit disorder.

- **Antipsychotics:** Treat psychotic symptoms, such as delusions, hallucinations, and schizophrenia.

- **Mood stabilizers:** Treat bipolar disorder and mood swings.

How psychiatric medications work

Psychiatric medications are psychoactive drugs that act on chemical messengers in our body called **neurotransmitters** and **hormones.**[23] Neurotransmitters travel across junctions between two nerve cells called synapses, while hormones travel through the circulatory system from glands to target organs.

For example, chemical substances called Benzodiazepines (BZD) are known to enhance the effect of a neurotransmitter called gamma-aminobutyric acid (GABA). BZD is now one of the most common medications for treating anxiety.[24]

Almost all antidepressants used today are designed based on a hypothesis called *"the monoamine hypothesis of depression.*[25]*"*

Monoamines are a specific type of neurotransmitters that occur in virtually all vertebrates[26] Serotonin, Norepinephrine, and Dopamine are examples of monoamines.

The hypothesis postulates that a deficit of monoamine neurotransmitters is responsible for certain symptoms of depression such as lack of energy, attention, motivation, and pleasure.[27] Therefore, depressive symptoms could be improved by increasing the level of monoamine neurotransmitters, according to the hypothesis. The original concept was born in the 1950s, and it is still the primary design principle for antidepressants today.[28] It is important to remember that the hypothesis focuses on suppressing symptoms, not about curing the root cause of the symptoms.

Antidepressants are categorized by what monoamines they target, and how they affect them. Serotonin, Norepinephrine, and Dopamine are commonly targeted monoamines. Common antidepressant types are SSRI, SARI, SNRI, and NDRI. **SSRI** stands for Selective Serotonin Reuptake Inhibitor. **SARI** stands for Serotonin Antagonist and Reuptake Inhibitor. **SNRI** stands for Serotonin Norepinephrine Reuptake Inhibitor. And **NDRI** stands for Norepinephrine Dopamine Reuptake Inhibitor. As you notice, all these names begin with the names of neurotransmitters, followed by a phrase "reuptake inhibitor." What is reuptake inhibitor?

Reuptake is a phenomenon that occurs at neural synaptic cells".[26] When neurotransmitters flow from a transmitting side to a receiving side at synaptic cells, not all neurotransmitters pass through. Some of them are reabsorbed by the transmitting side without being received at the receiving side. This phenomenon is called reuptake. The idea of most common antidepressants is to inhibit reuptake at the transmitting side so that more neurotransmitters will flow to the receiving side, thereby increasing the level of monoamine neurotransmitters. That's what the "reuptake inhibitor" means. So, SSRI for example is a drug that attempts to inhibit the reuptake phenomenon for Serotonin. SNRI and NDRI attempt to inhibit reuptake of Serotonin and Norepinephrine (SN) and Norepinephrine and Dopamine (ND), respectively.

Since these explanations sound legitimate, you may think that the antidepressants are the cure for mental health. That's not the case, unfortunately. First of all, the monoamine hypothesis is still a hypothesis and has not been proven yet, and the exact mechanism of how the reuptake inhibitor works is not well understood.[28] Some new forms of antidepressants do not act on monoamines, instead acting on different neurotransmitters called glutamate. They have been under study in recent years,[29] but scientists are still searching for an effective medication mechanism for depression.

The most important point to remember here is that the **antidepressants are designed to suppress the depressive symptoms**, not designed to cure the illness or root cause. Think about Tylenol, for example. It's a common medication to reduce fever or reduce minor pain. It suppresses the symptoms of fever or pain, but it does not cure the underlying illness of flu or arthritis. Antidepressants and all other psychiatric medications are symptom suppressants, a measure to relieve discomfort for patients, not a cure for the illness.

Side effects

The risks of psychiatric medications are well documented. Because each medication has variable efficacy and associated side effects, patients may need to try different medications before finding the one that improves their symptoms and causes less side effects.

The National Institute of Mental Health lists possible side effects of antidepressants:[22] *Nausea and vomiting, weight gain, diarrhea, sleepiness, suicidal thoughts, panic attacks, trouble sleeping, irritability and aggression, sexual problems.*

The following is a list of possible side effects of anti-anxiety medications:[22] *Nausea, blurred vision, headache, confusion, tiredness, nightmares, drowsiness, dizziness, difficulty thinking or remembering.*

Common psychiatric medications in the market

The table below shows the top 10 psychiatric medications prescribed in the US in 2013, identified by *PsychCentral*.[30] Further details of each drug can be found at the *National Alliance of Mental Illness* https://www.nami.org/ or MedlinePlus https://medlineplus.gov/ by typing a drug name in their search boxes.

Rank	Brand (Generic)	Main purpose	Type	U.S. Prescription
1	Xanax (Alprazolam)	Anxiety	Benzodiazepine	48.5 million
2	Zoloft (Sertraline)	Depression	SSRI	41.4 million
3	Celexa (Citalopram)	Depression	SSRI	39.4 million

Rank	Brand (Generic)	Main purpose	Type	U.S. Prescription
4	Prozac (Fluoxetine HCL)	Depression	SSRI	28.2 million
5	Ativan (Lorazepam)	Anxiety	Benzodiazepine	27.9 million
6	Desyrel (Trazodone HCL)	Depression	SARI	26.2 million
7	Lexapro (Escitalopram)	Depression	SSRI	24.9 million
8	Cymbalta (Duloxetine)	Depression	SNRI	18.6 million
9	Wellbutrin XL (Bupropion HCL XL)	Depression	NDRI	16.1 million

Rank	Brand (Generic)	Main purpose	Type	U.S. Prescription
10	Effexor ER (Venlafaxine HCL ER)	Depression	SNRI	15.8 million

Notice in this table that eight of the top ten medications are anti-depressants. Notice also that seven out of eight antidepressants target **Serotonin.** For anti-anxiety, Benzodiazepines (BZD) has been the primary substance for treatment.

Not in the table but commonly used medications for attention deficit disorders (ADD) include Vyvanse, Concerta, Amphetamine salts, and Methylphenidate. Abilify, Seroquel, Risperdal, and Zyprexa are used for bipolar disorders and schizophrenia. For panic disorders, the same anti-anxiety medications are commonly prescribed. Also, there are special types of medications for alcoholism treatment (Acamprosate, Naltrexone) and heroin detoxification (Methadone, Buprenorphine). Other diagnosed symptoms like obsessive compulsive disorder, post-traumatic stress disorder, and premenstrual dysphoric disorder are treated with the same medications used for the other major symptoms.[31]

Readers are encouraged to investigate the details of specific drugs, their intended use, and associated side effects. Reputable sources are listed below.

FDA https://www.fda.gov/

NIMH https://www.nimh.nih.gov/index.shtml

NAMI https://www.nami.org/

MedlinePlus https://medlineplus.gov/

Drugs.com   https://www.drugs.com/

MedicineNet   https://www.medicinenet.com/script/main/hp.asp

2.2. Psychiatric supplements

In the U.S., prescription and over-the-counter medications are regulated and must be approved by the Food and Drug Administration (FDA) to be marketed. However, there are chemical substances in the market that are not regulated by the FDA. They are called dietary supplements.

According to the FDA, dietary supplements are defined as follows:

"A dietary supplement is a product intended for ingestion that contains a 'dietary ingredient' intended to add further nutritional value to (supplement) the diet. A 'dietary ingredient' may be one, or any combination, of the following substances: a vitamin, a mineral, an herb or other botanical, an amino acid, a dietary substance for use by people to supplement the diet by increasing the total dietary intake, and a concentrate, metabolite, constituent, or extract."[32]

In other words, the FDA recognizes supplements as foods and therefore "does not have the authority to review dietary supplement products for safety and effectiveness before they are marketed."[33] Not being subject to the FDA regulation, it is no surprise that supplements are a big business. According to a study by the National Center for Health Statistics published in 2009, Americans spend $34 billion annually on complementary and alternative remedies, $7 billion on vitamin supplements, and 14.8 billion on non-vitamin, non-mineral, natural products (e.g. fish oil, glucosamine).[34]

Many supplements are marketed for mental health. The list below shows popular supplements for mental health, identified by Be Brain Fit.[35]

- DHA (Docosahexaenoic acid) (e.g., omega-3 fatty acid, fish oil)

- Citicoline

- Curcumin (active ingredient in turmeric)

- Acetylcarnitine (ALC)

- Phosphatidylserine (PS)

- Vinpocetine

- Alpha GPC

- Bacopa Monnieri

- Huperzine A

- Ginkgo Biloba

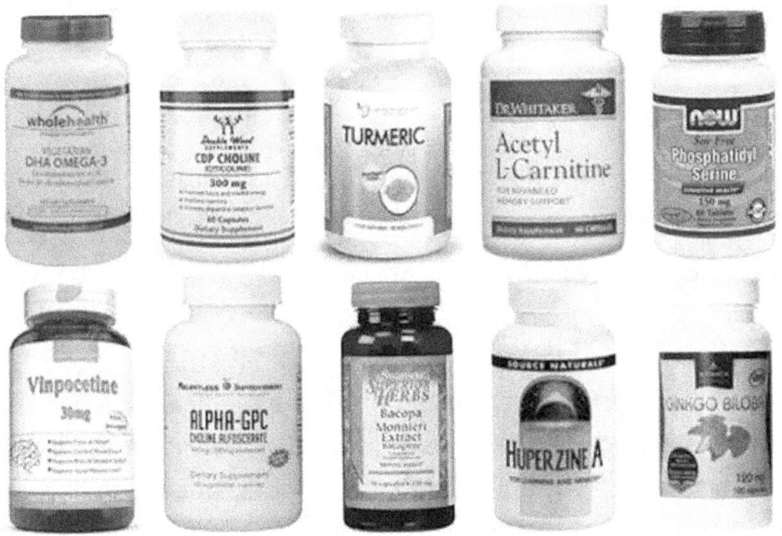

Figure 7. Popular supplements for mental health

Vitamins, minerals, and amino acids are also popular as supplements for mental health. The list below is from an article at *Everyday Health.*[36]

- Vitamin B-12

- Vitamin C

- Vitamin D

- Amino Acids

- Calcium

- Magnesium

- GABA

- Melatonin

- Probiotics

- SAM-e (S-adenosylmethionine)

2.3. Prescription process

Psychiatric medications are prescription drugs. So, who can prescribe them? They are:

1. **psychiatrists,**

2. **primary care doctors** or any physician with a valid medical license,

3. **physician's assistants,** and

4. **nurse practitioners.**

Psychologists in general cannot prescribe medications, except in some states, *e.g., Illinois, Louisiana, and New Mexico.*[37] Psychology is a diverse field with different types of specialties such as developmental psychology, forensic psychology, and sport psychology. Specialists who handle mental health in clinical environment are called clinical psychologists. They focus on psychiatric assessment and psychotherapies based on various psychology theories. Since they cannot prescribe medications, they will need to refer their clients to a physician if medication is deemed necessary. Psychiatrists, on the other hand, are trained in medicine. They perform psychiatric assessment, psychotherapies, and prescribe medications.

Psychiatric patient workflow

It helps to understand how health-care systems handle incoming patients with mental health issues. The flowchart below shows the process. There are three processing points of patient encounter where psychiatric medications can be prescribed:

1. initial assessment,

2. in-patient assessment, and

3. out-patient assessment.

Initial assessments are done by primary care physicians. In-patient and out-patient assessments are done by psychiatric specialists (clinical psychologists or psychiatrists).

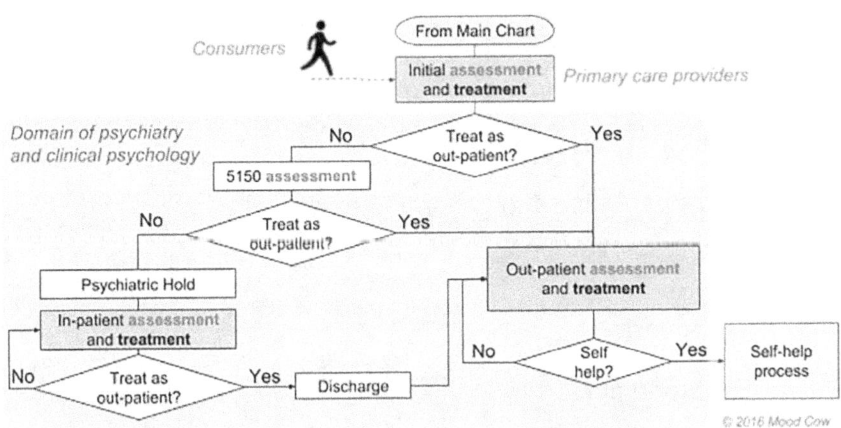

Figure 8. Clinical workflow of mental health patients' treatment

Complete psychiatric evaluation

Before prescribing medications, your doctor needs to perform a thorough psychiatric evaluation. According to the guidelines published by the American Psychiatric Association, evaluations are complex, time-consuming, and "involve a systematic consideration of the broad domains described in the guideline and vary in scope and intensity."[38] The domains described in the guideline are listed below.

- Reason for the evaluation

- History of the present illness

- Past psychiatric history

- History of alcohol and other substance use

- General medical history

- Developmental, psychosocial, and sociocultural history

- Occupational and military history

- Legal history

- Family history

- Review of systems

- Physical examination

- Mental status examination

  - Appearance and general behavior

  - Motor activity

  - Speech

  - Mood and affect

  - Thought processes

  - Thought content

  - Perceptual disturbances

  - Sensorium and cognition

  - Insight

  - Judgment Functional assessment

- Diagnostic tests

- Information derived from the interview process

These guidelines illustrate the complexity and resource-intensive nature of psychiatric assessment. Unfortunately, under the current protocol in primary care settings, **primary care physicians have no time or training to perform such lengthy assessment**. Therefore, they resort to the use of **quick screening tools, i.e. PHQ-9 and GAD-7** (see Chapter 1, Figures 3 and 4). Because of this, in the current primary care setting, a quick screening of symptoms directly results in a decision to medicate the patient, without understanding the underlying cause and stressors. Eighty percent of antidepressants were prescribed by non-psychiatric specialists without psychiatric diagnosis.[21] This is the reason why medication is the first choice of treatment in health care, not because of its efficacy.

References

19. Nesse RM. and Berridge KC. Psychoactive Drug Use in Evolutionary Perspective. *Science*. Vol.278. pp.63-66. 3 October 1997. https://www.ncbi.nlm.nih.gov/pubmed/9311928

20. Pratt LA, Brody DJ, Gu Q. Antidepressant use in persons aged 12 and over: United States, 2005–2008. NCHS data brief. National Center for Health Statistics. 2011. https://www.cdc.gov/nchs/products/databriefs/db283.htm

21. Mojtabai R. Olfson M. Proportion Of Antidepressants Prescribed Without A Psychiatric Diagnosis Is Growing. *Health Affairs*. 2011;30(8):1434-1442. https://www.ncbi.nlm.nih.gov/pubmed/21821561

22. National Institute of Mental health. Mental Health Medications. Retrieved from https://www.nimh.nih.gov/health/topics/mental-health-medications/index.shtml

23. National Institute on Drug Abuse. Impacts of Drugs on Neurotransmission. Retrieved from https://www.drugabuse.gov/news-events/nida-notes/2017/03/impacts-drugs-neurotransmission

24. MedicineNet.com. Oral Benzodiazepines Names, Side Effects, and Addiction. Retrieved from https://www.medicinenet.com/benzodiazepines_sleep-inducing-oral/article.htm

25. Delgado PL. Depression: The Case for a Monoamine Deficiency. *Journal of Clinical Psychiatry*. 61(suppl 6):7-11. 2000. https://www.ncbi.nlm.nih.gov/pubmed/10775018

26. Sotnikova TD and Gainetdinov RR. Octopamine and Other Monoamines in Invertebrates. *Encyclopedia of Neuroscience*. Academic Press. pp.9-15. 2009. https://www.sciencedirect.com/science/article/pii/B978008045046901158X

27. Lopez-Munoz F. and Alamo C. Monoaminergic neurotransmission: the history of the discovery of antidepressants from 1950s until today. Curr Pharm Des. 2009;15(14):1563-86. https://www.ncbi.nlm.nih.gov/pubmed/19442174

28. Hirschfeld RM. History and evolution of the monoamine hypothesis of depression. *Journal of Clinical Psychiatry*. 61 Suppl 6: 4–6. 2000. https://www.ncbi.nlm.nih.gov/pubmed/10775017

29. Hillhouse TM. and Porter JH. A brief history of the development of antidepressant drugs: From monoamines to glutamate. *Experimental and Clinical Psychopharmacology*, 23(1), 1-21. 2015. https://www.ncbi.nlm.nih.gov/pmc/articles/PMC4428540/

30. Grohol J. Psych Central. Top 25 Psychiatric Medication Prescriptions for 2013. Retrieved on May 12, 2016. Retrieved from https://psychcentral.com/lib/top-25-psychiatric-medication-prescriptions-for-2013/

31. Baldwin DS. et. al. Evidence-based pharmacological treatment of anxiety disorders, post-traumatic stress disorder and obsessive-compulsive disorder: A revision of the 2005 guidelines from the British Association for Psychopharmacology. *Journal of Psychopharmacology*. Volume: 28. Issue: 5. Pages: 403-439. 2014. http://journals.sagepub.com/doi/abs/10.1177/0269881114525674?journalCode=jopa

32. US Food and Drug Administration. FDA 101: Dietary Supple-

ments. Retrieved from https://www.fda.gov/ForConsumers/ConsumerUpdates/ucm050803.htm

33. US Food and Drug Administration. Dietary Supplements: What You Need to Know. Retrieved from https://www.fda.gov/Food/DietarySupplements/UsingDietarySupplements/ucm109760.htm

34. Nahin RL. Barnes PM. Stussman BJ. Bloom B. Costs of Complementary and Alternative Medicine (CAM) and Frequency of Visits to CAM Practitioners: United States, 2007. National health statistics reports; no 18. Hyattsville, MD: National Center for Health Statistics. 2009. https://nccih.nih.gov/sites/nccam.nih.gov/files/nhsrn18.pdf

35. Alban D. Be Brain Fit. Top 15 Brain Supplements for a Mental Edge. Retrieved on May 12, 2016 from https://bebrainfit.com/brain-supplements/

36. Borchard T. Everyday Health. 12 Patient-Approved Natural Supplements for Depression. Retrieved on May 12, 2016 from https://www.everydayhealth.com/columns/therese-borchard-sanity-break/patient-approved-natural-supplements-depression/

37. Mental Health America. Types of Mental Health Professionals. Retrieved on May 12, 2016 from http://www.mentalhealthamerica.net/types-mental-health-professionals

38. Practice Guideline for the Psychiatric Evaluation of Adults. Second Edition. American Psychiatric Association. June 2006. https://psychiatryonline.org/doi/pdf/10.1176/appi.books.9780890426760

CHAPTER 3

PSYCHOTHERAPIES

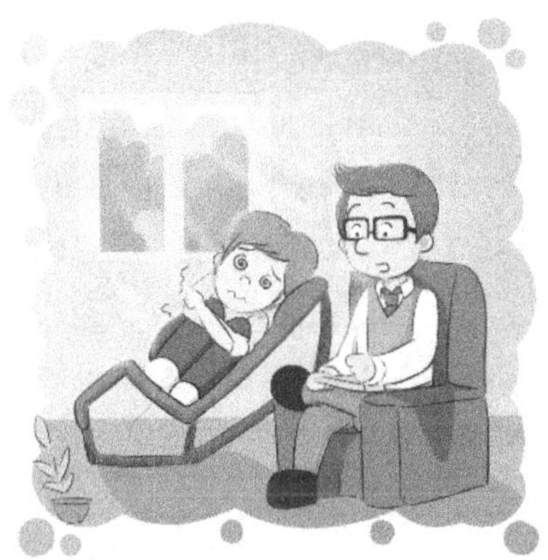

3.1. Psychotherapy overview

ACCORDING TO THE American Psychological Association (APA), "Psychotherapy is a collaborative treatment based on the relationship between an individual and a psychologist."[39] It is a type of treatment to control mental and behavioral problems through a series of conversations between a therapist and a patient. Conversations are structured differently based on the underlying theories informing them. Many theories exist, and so do therapists and therapies.

Efficacy of psychotherapy

Psychology theories are built on philosophical constructs; therefore, it is intrinsically difficult to compare and analyze how effective they are. In general, the efficacy depends on the patient's condition and level of effort, how the methods are administered, and the therapist's skill and experience.

In the U.S., the only mechanism to regulate the quality of therapy is by licensing. The exact licensing requirements vary by state. A person doesn't have to have a psychologist degree to perform psychotherapy. In California, for example, a person who is licensed by the Medical Board of California, California Board of Psychology, or California Board of Behavioral Sciences can practice psychotherapy. In addition, nurses, social workers, and interns who register and meet certain conditions can also perform psychotherapy or counseling within the state, according to California Code.[40]

With the rapid expansion of therapy services available over the phone, Internet, or even through a mobile app, you may see therapists outside of your state or country. Consumers should be aware of varying degrees of qualification and quality from people who call themselves "therapists."

3.2. Types of therapies

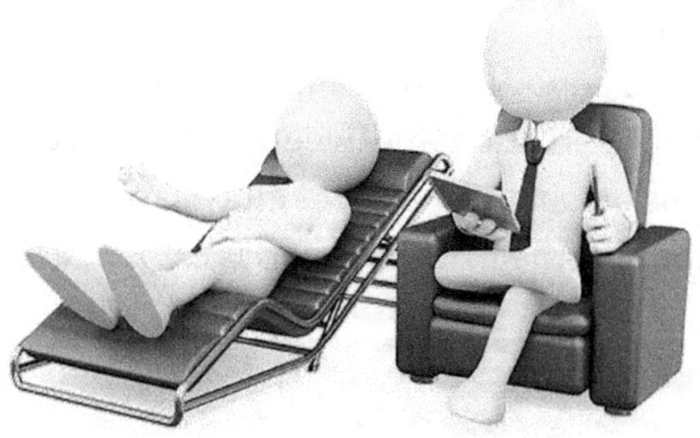

A large variety of approaches exist in psychotherapy. Wikipedia, for example, identifies over 150 psychotherapies. Unfortunately, it is extremely difficult for consumers to figure out which approach works best for their needs. The distinction among approaches is blurry and is differentiated mostly by philosophical roots, not necessarily by consumer needs.

According to the American Psychological Association, approaches to psychotherapy fall into five broad categories.[41]

- Psychoanalysis and psychodynamic therapies: Based on a theory about changing thoughts by exploring unconscious meanings.

- Behavior therapy: Based on a theory about changing behavior by learning normal and abnormal behaviors.

- Cognitive therapy: Based on a theory about changing thoughts by learning normal and abnormal thoughts.

- Humanistic therapy: Based on a theory about respect and human capacity to make rational choices.

- Integrative or holistic therapy: Blending elements from different approaches.

This is still a philosophical categorization and is not practical or useful for consumers. Instead of relying on dogmatic views, consumers should look at the practical purposes and features of psychotherapies. For that reason, I identified five therapy types:

- **Cognitive behavioral therapy** (CBT),

- **Dialectical behavior therapy** (DBT),

- **Interpersonal psychotherapy** (IPT),

- **Creative arts therapies** (CAT), and

- **Family counseling.**

3.2.1. Cognitive Behavioral Therapy (CBT)

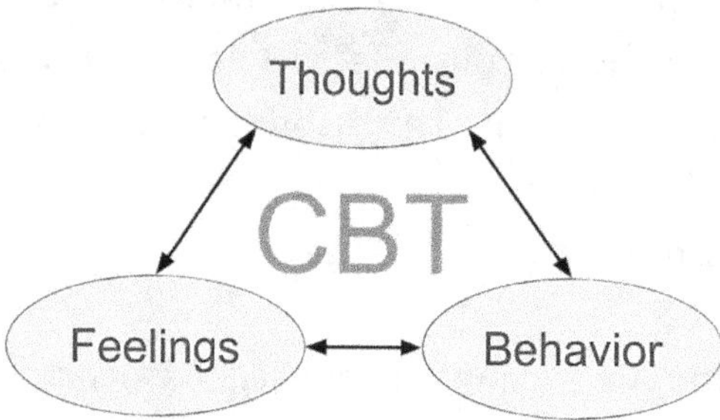

CBT is not a single therapy method; rather, it is a class of therapies that share the same principle — *changes in thoughts can improve feelings and behavior*. The exact procedure varies among therapists, but the general features can be highlighted as follows:

- CBT is **goal-oriented**. The process begins by identifying problematic feelings and behaviors.

- CBT is **collaborative**. The therapist and patient work together to find appropriate skills necessary to solve the problem.

- CBT **requires homework**. The patient must work to learn the necessary skills.

- CBT is **short-term**. Therapy may end in less than 20 sessions or 5 months.

CBT is commonly used to treat a variety of mental conditions such as depression, anxiety, addiction, and dependence. The good news for consumers is that CBT is prevalent, and many online resources are available to learn more about it.

PsychCentral is a good starting place for learning about the basics of CBT
https://psychcentral.com/lib/in-depth-cognitive-behavioral-therapy

Wikipedia shows a list of CBT therapies. https://en.wikipedia.org/wiki/List_of_cognitive%E2%80%93behavioral_therapies

Explore with search keyword "cognitive behavioral therapy."

3.2.2. Dialectical Behavior Therapy (DBT)

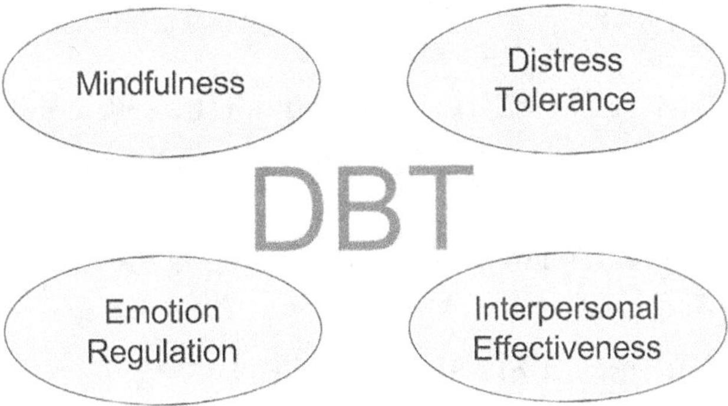

DBT is a special type of CBT, originally developed by psychologist Marsha M. Linehan in the 1980s, to treat suicidal individuals diagnosed with borderline personality disorder. Since then, DBT has been used to treat a variety of conditions, including depression, substance dependence, and post-traumatic stress disorder.

As the term "dialectical" implies, DBT emphasizes the integration of opposite strategies: **acceptance and change**. While change is the core strategy of CBT, DBT recognizes that some patients do not respond well to the forced change that CBT demands. DBT integrates the concept of acceptance from Buddhism as a way of preparation and acclimatization for patients to make progress toward eventual changes.

DBT uniquely teaches four sets of behavioral skills:

- **Mindfulness:** Learn to be aware of the present moment.

- **Distress tolerance:** Learn to tolerate pain in difficult situations.

- **Emotion regulation:** Learn to think differently.

- **Interpersonal effectiveness:** Learn to communicate with self-respect.

The good news for consumers is that there are numerous online resources available to learn more about DBT.

The Linehan Institute has the most authoritative information about DBT. http://behavioraltech.org/resources/whatisdbt.cfm

Explore with search keyword "dialectical behavior therapy."

3.2.3. Interpersonal Psychotherapy

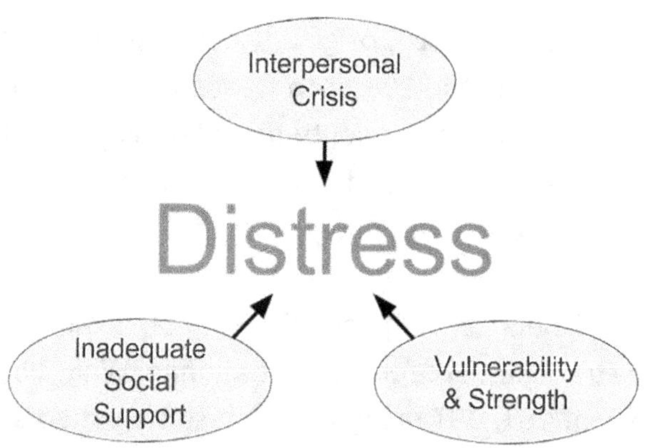

IPT is a time-limited therapy that focuses on interpersonal issues. It aims to improve symptoms, interpersonal functioning, and social support in 6~20 sessions. It was originally developed in the 1970s by Gerald Klerman, Myrna Weissman, and Eugene Paykel to treat depression. Since then, IPT has been used for a variety of conditions, populations, and settings.

IPT appears to be more approachable than CBT for young people and older adults because it emphasizes relationships and requires less homework than CBT. In addition, IPT uses less technical words than other psychotherapies, making it more accessible to wider populations.

WebMD has good, easy to digest information about IPT. https://www.webmd.com/depression/guide/ interpersonal-therapy-for-depression#1

Explore with search keyword "interpersonal psychotherapy."

3.2.4. Creative Arts Therapies (CAT)

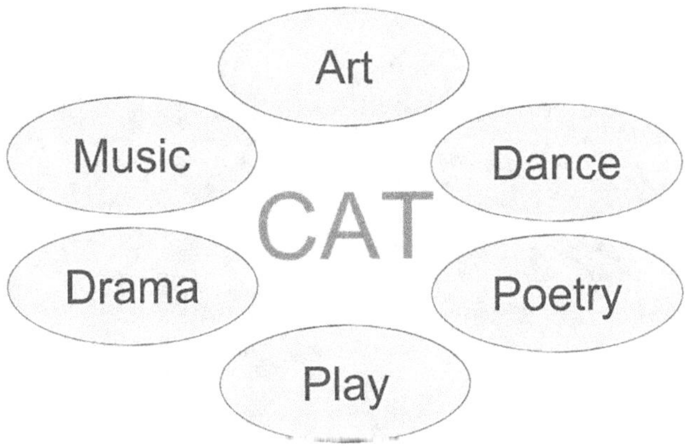

CAT (also called Expressive Therapies) is an umbrella term for a group of therapies that use creative, expressive, artistic activities as a remedy for mental conditions. Based on the principle that creative expression and imagination improve awareness of the body, feelings, and thoughts, CAT therapists use imagery, music, dance, movement, drama, poetry, storytelling, and visual arts in an integrated way to help patients heal or foster growth.

While most psychotherapies utilize a cognitive mode of action for healing, CAT is unique in its focus on sensory and physical modes. Consumers may find CAT a good alternative to classic talk therapies like CBT and IPT. The International Expressive Arts Therapy Association and National Coalition of Creative Arts

Therapies Associations are promoting CAT worldwide and in the US, respectively.

Psychology Today has a good summary of CAT. https://www.psychologytoday.com/us/blog/arts-and-health/201406/ creative-arts-therapy-and-expressive-arts-therapy

Explore with search keyword "creative arts therapy."

3.2.5. Family Counseling

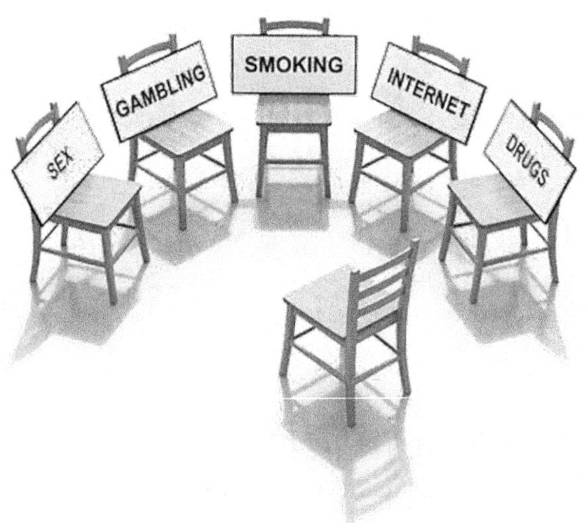

Family counseling (or family therapy) is an important branch of psychotherapy that emphasizes relationships as an important factor in mental health. Although family counseling has a long history in various cultures, the contemporary therapeutic form originates from child guidance and marriage counseling in the early 20th century. Since then, the field evolved beyond the traditional family to include relationships among people who are not related by blood or marriage.

Like CBT and other psychotherapies, the exact method and procedure for family counseling differs among therapists. Some common features are:

Short-term: The number of sessions may be between 5 and 20.

All members meet: Members of the family (or group) meet at the same time to observe habitual interaction patterns.

Less focus on cause-effect analysis: Rather than blaming individuals, therapists and patients work together to find ways to better the situation.

Consumers may find family counseling an important resource to resolve issues at home, work, or school to avoid serious consequences if left unresolved.

Mayo Clinic has a good summary of family counseling.

https://www.mayoclinic.org/tests-procedures/family-therapy/about/pac-20385237

Explore with search keyword "family counseling."

References

39. American Psychological Association. Understanding psychotherapy and how it works. Retrieved on May 12, 2016 from http://www.apa.org/helpcenter/understanding-psychotherapy.aspx

40. California Business and Professions Code (BPC), Division 2 Healing Arts [500 - 4999.129], Chapter 14. Social Workers [4991 - 4998.5]. Retrieved on May 12, 2016 from http://leginfo.legislature.ca.gov/faces/codes.xhtml

41. American Psychological Association. Different approaches to psychotherapy. Retrieved on May 12, 2016 from http://www.apa.org/topics/therapy/psychotherapy-approaches.aspx

Summary of Part 1

What we learned in this section

- Inadequacy of current mental health care is well evidenced in scientific literature. Treatment options are limited, efficacy is questionable, and the healthcare process is not aligned with the demands and delicate, complex natures of mental health.

- In the meantime, indiscriminate prescription of psychiatric medications remains prevalent, and the unregulated supplement industry is booming.

- Importance of prevention is acknowledged in public health, but no effective methodology is established.

What this means for you

- Doctors are an important resource for your mental health, but you need to be cautious with treatment options they offer, especially medications. Avoid taking psychiatric medi cations prescribed by primary care doctors unless a qualified psychologist or psychiatrist performs a complete psychiatric assessment.

- Not all medications are the same. Read all fine prints and ask questions about the intended use and side effects. Work with your doctor to set clear, reasonable expectations for outcomes, and always discuss options other than medications if possible.

- Not all psychotherapies are the same. Before engaging with a therapy, ask questions to understand the underlying theories and method. The quality and benefits of therapies depend on the level of your effort too. Work with your therapists to set clear, reasonable expectations for outcomes, and make sure that you understand what you need to do to achieve the goal.

PART 2

SYNTHESIS

The second part of this book is about building a solution to the problems identified in Part 1. Chapter 4 presents the principles of mental care and a framework of mental care processes. Chapter 5 explores the risk and protective factors for mental well-being, and presents a systematic method to collect and analyze data. Chapter 6 presents the concept of mental care curriculum for early childhood education.

THE PRINCIPLES OF MENTAL CARE

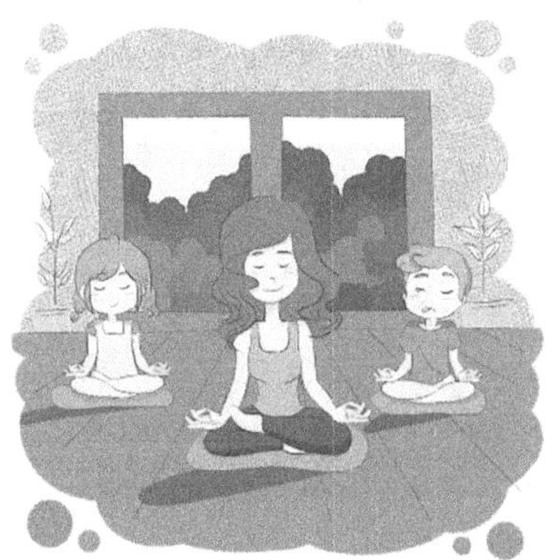

FEELINGS ARE THE most important factor in our well-being. Since everyone has good days and bad days, everyone should know how to perform routine mental care, just like dental care. To promote a systematic approach to mental health prevention and maintenance, this chapter establishes the foundations of mental care from a systems science perspective. It starts with four principles.

4.1. The principles

1. All feelings are natural and acceptable, but poor behavior is not.

Humans are emotional creatures. It is natural to feel sad, anxious, angry, or to experience any feelings under various circumstances. All feelings are natural no matter how strong; therefore, all feelings are acceptable. Everyone has good days and bad days, and everyone has feelings. You are not alone.

While feelings are invisible to others, they are often reflected in behavior. Humans are social creatures, and we don't exist alone. Our social standard requires that everyone knows how to act given moral and ethical considerations. Behavior outside of confines is considered poor, and poor behavior is often harmful to oneself and others. Regardless of the types and strength of feelings, poor behavior is not acceptable.

Understanding this principle is an important part of our mental care. If, for any reason, you cannot manage your feelings and behavior, you should consider this as a medical condition and seek help from your health-care provider for intervention.

2. There are risk and protective factors in life that influence your mental well-being.

Everyone is different, genetically, neurologically, and environmentally. Everyone reacts to influencers differently. Even the same person may react differently depending on their body's biochemical balance at that moment. There are risk factors and protective factors in life that influence your mental well-being negatively or positively. In principle, we want to maximize the protective factors while minimizing the risk factors. Understanding these influencers is an important part of your mental care.

3. Mental care is an iterative process.

Wellness is a process. A process is not a thing that you can touch, or an idea that you dream about. A process is a series of actions you purposefully take to achieve a desirable state over time.

For example, consider dental care. No matter how many toothbrushes or how much toothpaste you may have, if you don't properly brush your teeth with them, it doesn't help. Mental care is the same. It's your awareness and actions that matter the most. That's the process.

A good process is one that continuously improves over time. It is not a good process if you keep changing your actions without making improvement. To have a good process, you need a system to check its effectiveness and make necessary adjustments for improvement, and do this iteratively.

Iteration means the repetition of a process. At each iteration, you take your preventive action, check its effectiveness, make an adjustment if necessary, and repeat the cycle. The quality of iteration makes mental care a good, effective process.

4. Medications and therapies are not the primary tools for mental care.

Despite common beliefs, medications and therapies are not the only tool options for mental care. There are six modes of treatment: sensory, biochemical, cognitive, social, spiritual, and physical.

- **Sensory mode:** Seeing, hearing, smelling, tasting, touching, or sensing of motion can help stimulate, relax, or regulate your needs. For example, nature, art, music, sound and voice, touching fabric, plush toys, feeling motions, wind, massages, aromas, food and beverages — they can all stimulate you, relax you, or help improve your condition. This is probably the most instantly gratifying mode of mental care treatment, but the effect may be limited or short-term.

- **Biochemical mode:** Sunlight, hydration, nutritional intake, medications, and supplements all have a direct impact on the chemical balance in your body. Alcoholic beverages and sweet snacks are not a positive biochemical substance because of their negative influence on your chemical balance. They should be considered a sensory mode — quick, short-term relief.

- **Cognitive mode:** Language and thoughts are the primary tool of this mode. For example, reading books, writing in journals, conversing with counselors are some of the many cognitive activities for self-help treatment.

- **Social mode:** Being in touch with friends, family, pets, or people in general can be stimulating, relaxing, and often helpful for regulation. Stress can arise in a social environment, but social relationships can also be a good remedy.

- **Spiritual mode:** Meditation and praying can be an important self-help mode, especially for regulation. Certain activities at churches or temples may offer additional social, sensory, and physical options.

- **Physical mode:** Physical activities can help stimulate, relax, or regulate your needs. Gardening, craft works, cooking, singing, playing musical instruments, dancing, golf, walking, exercising, stretching, deep breathing — the list is endless. This mode is favored, as it combines aspects of the sensory, biochemical, cognitive, social, and spiritual modes.

The common tools of choice by health-care providers are the biochemical mode (i.e. psychiatric medications) and the social and cognitive modes (i.e. psychotherapies). A variety of elements exist within each mode, as well as any combination of them, that would work for specific needs, preferences, and circumstances. It is important to know that there are choices other than drugs and therapies.

4.2. Mental care processes

Based on the principles, we can construct a systematic method for mental care.

4.2.1. System to determine when to seek medical help

First, based on the first principle, we want to build a system to define the role of health care and the responsibility of self, and use it as a tool to determine when to seek medical help. The system consists of three tests: mental capacity test, mental crisis test, and mental self-care test, as illustrated in the flowchart (Figure 9).

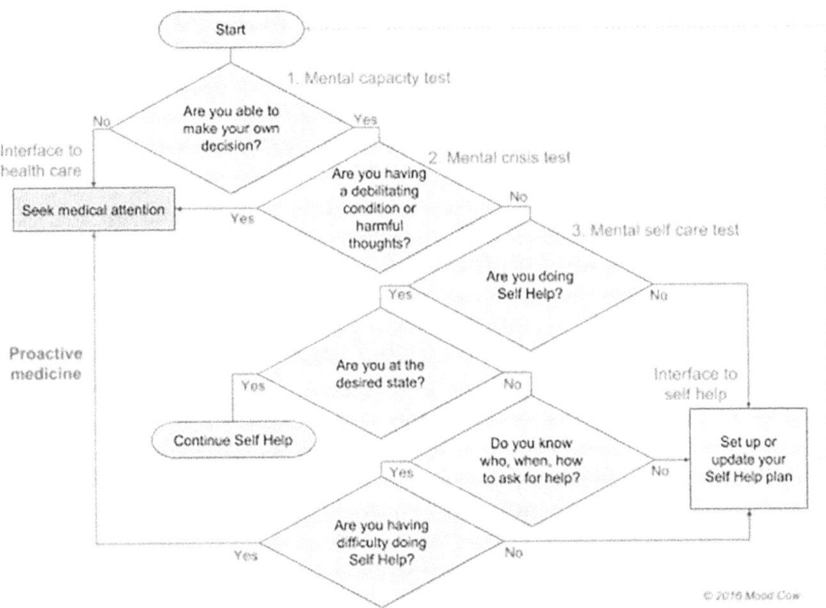

Figure 9. A systematic tool to determine when to seek medical help

Mental capacity test

If you are unable to make your own decisions, you need **medical attention.**

If you are able to make your own decision, proceed to take the mental crisis test.

Mental crisis test

If you are experiencing a debilitating condition or having harmful thoughts, you need **medical attention.**

If not, proceed to take the mental self-care test.

Mental self-care test

If you are not doing self-help, you need to set up a plan of self-help. Self-help is a goal-oriented, iterative process to reach and remain at a desired state. Self-help does **not** mean that you have to do everything by yourself; instead, you recognize your responsibility to create positive, routine actions for yourself.

If you are doing self-help, and if you are at a desired state, continue your current self-help routine. A desired state is where you are taking positive, routine actions, continuing the iterative process on your own, AND you know when, how, and who to ask for help when necessary.

If you are doing self-help but not achieving a desired state, and if you don't know when, how, and who to ask for help, identify and use the help resource.

If you are having difficulty carrying out a self-help process for any reason, you need to **seek medical attention.**

4.2.2. Self-help process

The third principle states that mental care is a process, a series of actions. A good mental care process improves over time by planning, doing, checking, and adjusting the series of actions, and by repeating the cycle. A desired mental care system is one that promotes such iterative process improvement, as illustrated in the flowchart.

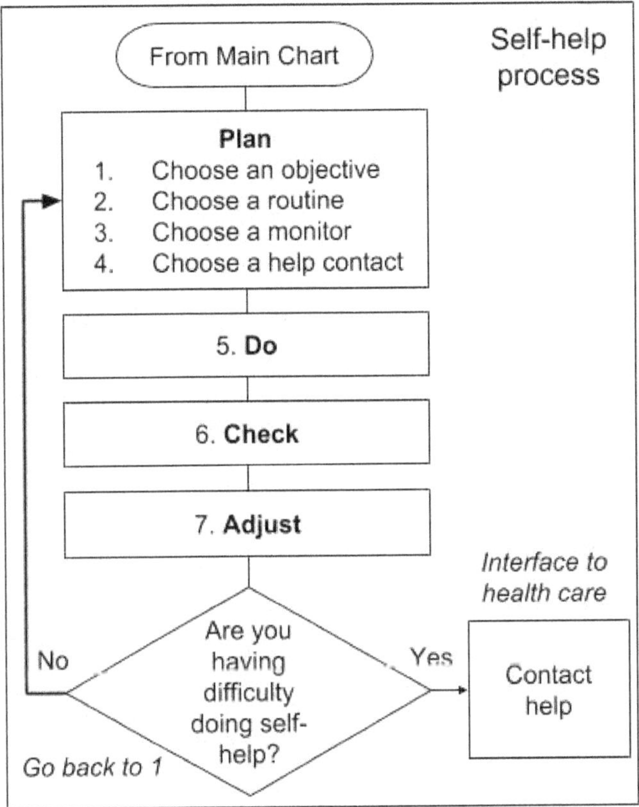

Figure 10. Iterative self-help process flowchart

Step 1: Choose an objective

Self-help begins with a plan, and setting a goal is the first, most important step. Principled mental care singles in on three objectives:

Stimulation: To increase energy or motivation, activate new interests, and invigorate life experiences.

Relaxation: To calm down, relax, and deactivate nervousness.

Regulation: To solve a specific problem or improve certain conditions such as insomnia, stress, anxiety, depression, or dealing with emotionally difficult times.

The first step in self-help is to ask yourself what you think you need to achieve right now: relaxation, stimulation, or regulation. For example, if you feel exhausted, anxious, nervous, upset, angry, or too worried, you may need to relax yourself. If you feel bored, depressed, or uninterested in anything, you may need to stimulate yourself.

While relaxation and stimulation may help your symptoms for a while, they don't necessarily solve underlying problems. If your condition bothers you quite a bit or is long-lasting, you may need to make problem-solving — in other words, regulation — your objective.

Regulation is different from relaxation and stimulation in that problem-solving requires you to think beyond your symptoms and how you are feeling. You need to think about what may be making you feel certain ways, how/why these things are affecting you, and what may help you cope with problems to make you feel better again.

Everyone has moments and special circumstances, and we all have to deal with them somehow. The principled framework helps you become aware of what you need to do and encourages you to do it.

Step 2: Choose a routine

Once you are aware of what you want to achieve, you need to think about how to achieve it. Principled mental care calls for a simple, routine action that you can do easily and consistently on a daily basis. Just as you brush your teeth every night for dental care or apply moisturizer after a shower for skin care, we want a simple routine for mental care.

You can choose a routine from any of the six modes of action for mental care: sensory, biochemical, cognitive, social, spiritual, and physical modes.

Sensory mode. Listening to music, smelling soothing aromas, looking out a scenery or artwork, touching soft fabrics. They are all examples of mental care in sensory mode. The effect may be short-term but it is the easiest and instantly gratifying routine.

Biochemical mode. Soaking up the sunlight, drinking water, eating nutritious food. They are effective routines that positively affect your biochemical balance in your body. Be cautious with medications, supplements, alcohol, and sweet snacks, because they all have side effects.

Cognitive mode. Reading books, writing in journals, vocalizing your feelings. These activities with language and thoughts are good mental care routine in cognitive mode. Conversing with a therapist, if you have one, is also a cognitive routine.

Social mode. Hanging out with friends, families, and pets is a rewarding mental care in social mode. Be cautious when tensions arise in social relationships, especially in digital communications.

Spiritual mode. Meditation, praying, attending faith-based activities have been an important mental care routine for centuries. Also, try giving kind words to people and helping out people in need. This adds a social mode to your routine and is very rewarding.

Physical mode. Any activity that moves your body can be a rewarding mental care routine. Walking, dancing, stretching, biking, gardening, cooking, singing, playing a musical instrument. Many physical activities combine sensory, biochemical, cognitive, social, and spiritual modes. One of the best mental care routine is deep breathing.

Step 3: Choose a monitor

Imagine a diet plan without a scale. How would you know if you are losing or gaining weight? You wouldn't. The same applies to mental care. You need a way to monitor your condition to know if you are achieving your objective.

Unlike body weight or temperature, mental condition is not easily measurable in numbers. Fortunately, there is a time-tested method that works for mental care: a mood diary. Simply writing down your mood in a notebook as part of a routine helps you improve your awareness and gain insight into your well-being. For those who prefer a more convenient method of journaling, there are an increasing number of mobile applications that are specifically designed to keep a record of your mood. You can find them by using keywords "mood diary" on your mobile app store.

Step 4: Choose a help contact

The last step of your self-help planning is to identify your primary support. If you need help, who do you call? How do you reach that person? Traditionally, such support used to be friends and family members. If you have someone in your family or friend group you can trust and rely on to call anytime, anywhere, for any reason, then great. Keep that in your record and use it.

If you can't think of anyone, don't worry. Use your health-care provider. Have a phone number of your primary care physician in case you need help. Phone calls to doctors don't cost anything, and doctors often know a variety of helpful services. Most healthcare systems these days have special resources allocated for a variety of emotional needs, such as group education and lifestyle coaching. They are reliable, trustworthy, resourceful, and most importantly, they care for you.

A very important resource in case of suicidal thoughts is the National Suicide Prevention Lifeline 1-800-273-8255 https://suicidepreventionlifeline.org/. They are available 24 hours every day for free and confidential support for people in distress.

Another important resource is the National Domestic Violence Hotline 1-800-799-7233 http://www.thehotline.org/. They are available 24 hours every day for free and confidential support. They also have an online chat service.

Make sure not to hesitate to use your help contact.

Step 5: Do it

It's time to actually do the routine you chose.

Step 6: Check it

Use your monitor to see how you are doing.

Step 7: Adjust it

Your initial choice of routine may or may not have worked. Adjust your routine if needed.

Step 8: Go back to Step 1

When you complete the first cycle, this is a good time to reach out to your help contact and share your insights about what worked, what didn't, and why. Schedule a meeting regularly — perhaps twice a year. Review and update your plan. Then, the cycle continues.

4.3. The role of therapies and medications in mental care

The fourth principle states that medications and therapies are not the primary tools for mental care. This is only valid when an individual is

1. Capable of making their own decisions (i.e. Satisfied the mental capacity test),

2. Not having a debilitating condition (i.e. Satisfied the mental crisis test), and

3. Not yet doing self-help or improving with the existing process (i.e. Failed the mental self-care test).

Self-help has limits. When an individual fails the mental capacity or crisis test, or has difficulty performing self-help, health-care providers become the primary resource for help. In this case, an ideal action would be a complete psychiatric evaluation, followed by therapies or medications, or both, directed by qualified healthcare providers. Caution is advised, however, as a major risk arises when medications are prescribed with only a quick assessment without thorough psychiatric evaluation.

Psychiatric medications in mental care

Psychiatric medications and supplements are a biochemical mode of treatment. As described in Chapter 2, medications work by biochemically controlling the functions of neurotransmitters and hormones. In other words, you are using drugs to suppress symptoms by directly affecting the brain functions without resolving any underlying root causes. Such treatment should only be necessary for disabling problems that cannot be regulated by other means of treatment.

For example, when an individual is suffering from hyper-anxiety and unable to think or talk, physicians may administer Benzodiazepines, such as Alprazolam or Lorazepam, to calm the symptom. This subsequently allows cognitive and social modes of treatment (i.e. counseling) to be effective.

Psychotherapies in principled mental care

Psychotherapies are **assisted self-help**. Therapies work because of the collaboration between a motivated patient and a skilled therapist. The collaboration is a social mode of mental care, with a variety of additional modes depending on the specific therapy types utilized.

For example, in the case of creative arts therapies, the patient will engage in sensory and physical modes. In dialectical behavior therapy, the patient will go through spiritual, sensory, cognitive, and physical modes. If the therapy is performed by a psychiatrist, a biochemical mode (psychiatric medications) may be administered in conjunction with psychotherapy.

The efficacy of psychotherapies depends on the therapist's skill, the patient's effort, collaboration, and the use of the modes of mental care. Therapy can be considered successful and complete if the patient is able to continue the self-help process without further supervision by the therapist.

Use a doctor as your support system

People often talk about support systems. They are typically referring to friends and family members who stand behind and help them by understanding their special circumstances. Doctors are also a good support resource. Your doctor understands the biomedical aspects of your health and can advise you with an objective view. Caution is advised, though, with physicians who overly rely on medications without understanding your situations, or performing a complete psychiatric assessment by a qualified psychologist or psychiatrist.

In order to maximize the value and minimize the risks of medications, work with your doctor to:

Discuss concerns you have, and stay connected and informed of any changes or developments in your condition.

Set clear, reasonable expectations for outcomes with any treatment plan.

Discuss options other than medications, and the risks of using medications.

Principled mental care as a unified framework

Principled mental care redefines self-help as the core of preventive mental care, encapsulating medications, therapies, and wellness services within the framework. By doing so, principled mental care encourages medical professionals, policy makers, health-care payers and providers, and researchers to come together to renovate mental health care as a unified system.

CHAPTER 5

RISK AND PROTECTIVE FACTORS

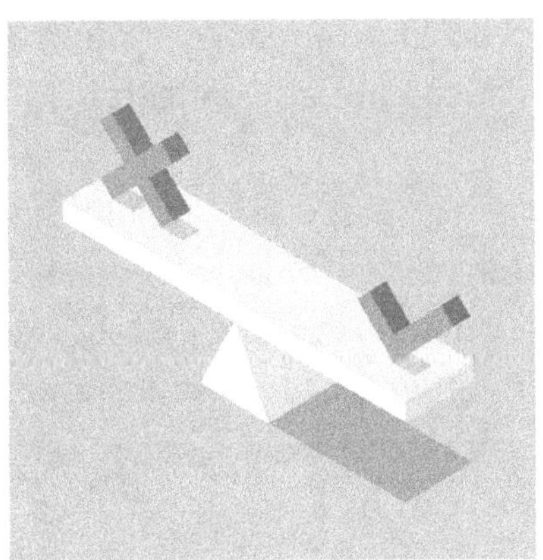

5.1. A systems approach to mental health

IN A TRADITIONAL health-care setting, we are seen by a doctor as a patient with a medical condition. The doctor listens to our verbal description of symptom complaints and asks us to fill in the assessment worksheets (i.e. PHQ-9 or GAD-7). The doctor then determines a treatment plan to control the symptom, typically by medication, psychotherapy, or both. This process is depicted in the figure below.

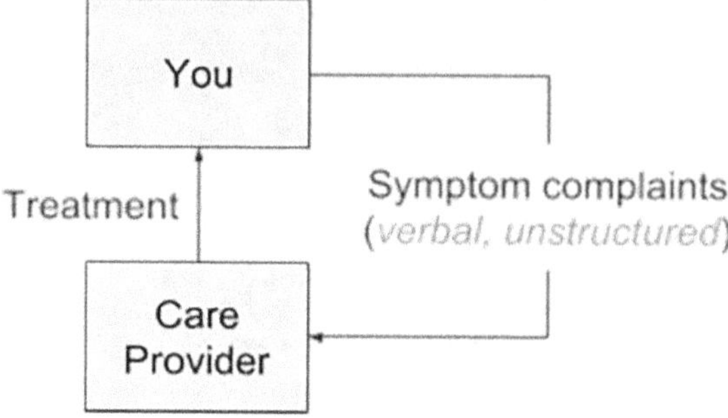

Figure 11. A system diagram of traditional mental health care

Unlike physical illness like flu where we can easily measure physical conditions, mental states are invisible and difficult to measure objectively. Diagnosis and treatment must therefore rely on what and how patients complain about their feelings and conditions. This subjective and qualitative nature of mental health treatment makes it not only difficult but also dangerous.

From a systems science perspective, mental states are unobservable under the current clinical environment, and any attempt from outside to regulate an unobservable system is prone to make the system unstable. In other words, treating a patient based solely on symptom complaints, and giving a patient an external influence such as medications, carries a risk of negative impact on system stability.

What is lacking in the traditional process is information. In principle, psychiatric evaluations exist for that purpose, by identifying many pieces of information about the patient. In reality, however, the required time, labor, and skills are not affordable under the current settings.

A systems view suggests an alternative. With the second principle of mental care, it is possible to improve the process by introducing

the risk and protective factors as inputs to the system. This view is illustrated in the system diagram below.

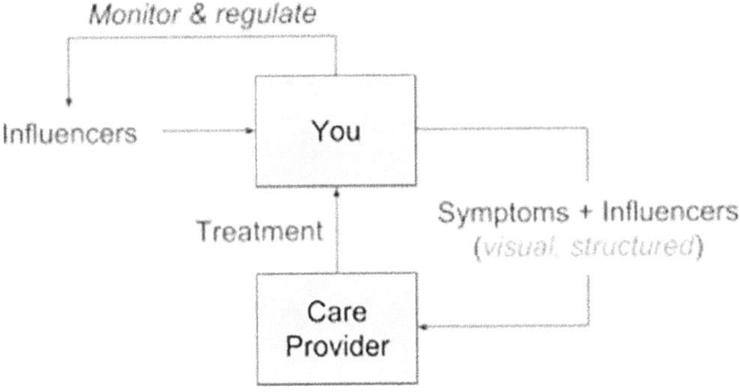

Figure 12. A system diagram of proposed mental health care

Here I introduce the term **influencers** to represent the risk and protective factors that influence our mental well-being. Negative influencers are the risk factors that affect our mental well-being negatively. Positive influencers are the protective factors that affect our mental well-being positively.

For example, suppose that you've been feeling a little sad for the past few days. You are not sure why you're feeling that way, but you can think of a few possible factors like, you are recovering from recent flu, it's been raining non-stop for a few days, and you can't go outside and exercise. These are the examples of negative influencers, the risk factors that affect your mental well-being negatively.

In the same example, you now try to think about what may make you feel better and overcome the negative feelings. Let's say that hanging out with your friends and listening to favorite music are two factors that help your mental well-being. These are examples of positive influencers, the protective factors that affect your mental well-being positively.

Think of influencers as balancers on a teeter-totter. Imagine yourself at the pivot point. On your right, you have negative influencers that make you feel down. On your left, you have positive influencers that make you feel up and balance against the weight of your negative influencers. A big negative worry factor may be balanced out with a few smaller but effective positive balancers.

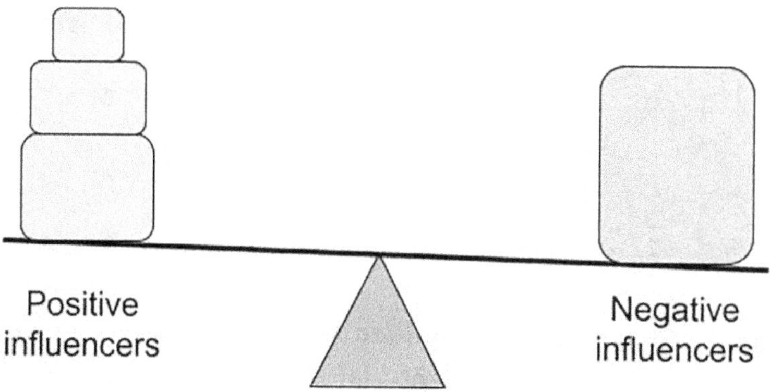

Figure 13. Positive and negative influencers as balancers

This approach has two benefits. First, it helps the care provider with additional information that relate to the patient's history and condition. Second, it helps the patient by providing a way to perform self-help by monitoring and regulating the influencers. Ideally, we want to keep track of influencers to enhance protective factors while minimizing risk factors.

Unfortunately, there is a problem in implementing this approach. There is no method available currently to represent and track influencers in health care. Here I propose a new method.

5.2. Structured influencers

Influencers are qualitative and subjective in nature. To make them quantitative and objective, we need to build a structure for them. Based on the World Health Organization's definition of health, we first construct three core dimensions of well-being: social, physical, and mental. We then assign external and internal orientations to each dimension, yielding six categorical dimensions.

- External social influencers (ESI)
- Internal social influencers (ISI)
- External physical influencers (EPI)
- Internal physical influencers (IPI)
- External mental influencers (EMI)
- Internal mental influencers (IMI)

Each influencer category has positive and negative orientation, yielding a total of twelve influencer categories.

1. External Social Influencers (ESI)

Social influencers are the social aspects of risk and protective factors. External social influencers involve social experience with the outside world. For example, positive ESI may include positive events In social life, good friends and family, and good living conditions. Negative ESI may include poor social life, stress at work, home or school, bereavement, and poor living conditions.

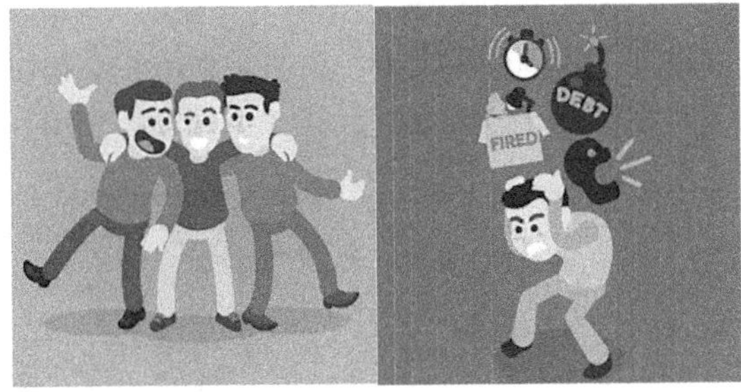

Figure 14. Positive and negative ESI

2. Internal Social Influencers

While external social influencers affect your mental well-being from outside social influence, internal social influencers affect you from inside of yourself, as in personality and social coping skills. For example, positive ISI may include positive "can do" attitudes, good social coping skills, confidence, and strong will power and determination to achieve a special goal. Negative ISI may include negative "can't do" attitudes, poor social coping skills, low self-esteem, and lack of confidence or motivation.

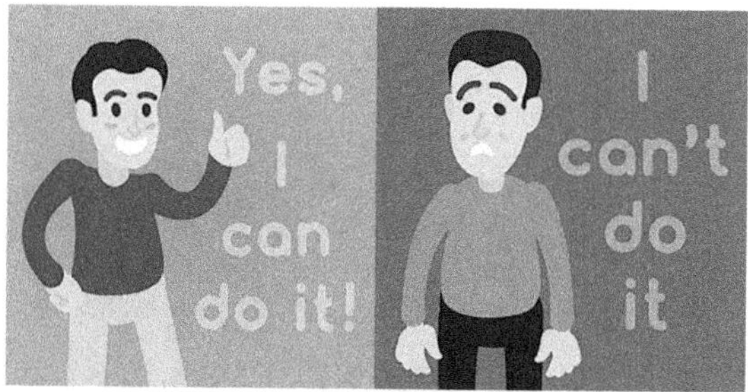

Figure 15. Positive and negative ISI

3. External Physical Influencers (EPI)

Physical influencers are the physical aspects of risk and protective factors. External physical influencers involve physical experience with the outside world. For example, positive EPI may include exercise, sports, music, good food, hobby, and nice weather. Negative EPI may include physical abuse and violence, substance abuse, medication that affects mood, poor nutrition, and poor weather.

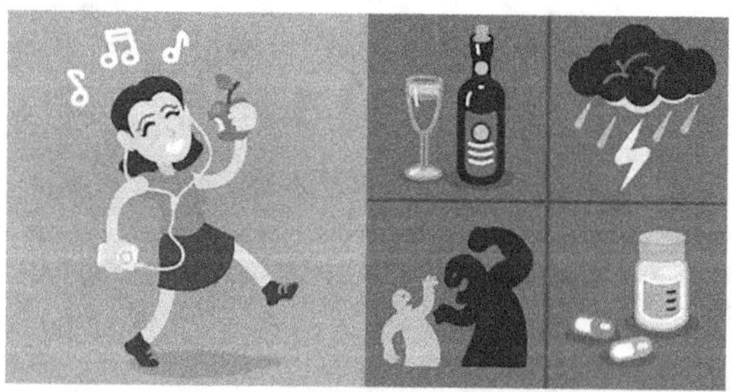

Figure 16. Positive and negative EPI

4. Internal Physical Influencers (IPI)

While external physical influencers affect your mental well-being from outside physical influence, internal physical influencers affect you from inside of yourself as in personal and internal physical conditions. For example, positive IPI may include good physical health and fitness. Negative IPI may include stress from illness, injury, or poor fitness, lack of sleep, or exhaustion.

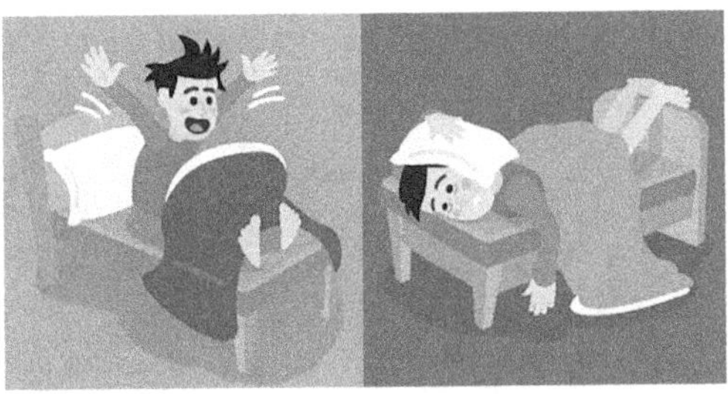

Figure 17. Positive and negative IPI

5. External Mental Influencers (EMI)

Mental influencers are the mental aspects of risk and protective factors. External mental influencers (EMI) involve mental and spiritual experiences with the outside world. For example, positive EMI may include goodwill help by someone or positive spiritual experience. Negative EMI may include emotional abuse, harassment, or bullying by someone.

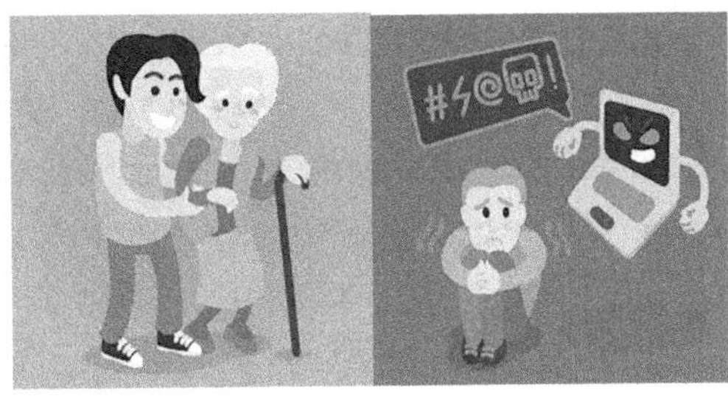

Figure 18. Positive and negative EMI

6. Internal Social Influencers (IMI)

While external mental influencers affect your mental well-being from outside mental influence, internal mental influencers (IMI) affect you from inside of yourself, as in personal and internal mental conditions. For example, positive IMI may include faith and spirituality. Negative IMI may include biological disorders that affect mood negatively.

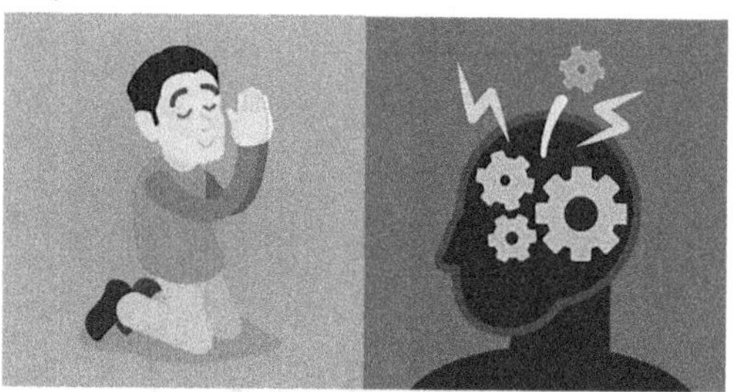

Figure 19. Positive and negative IMI

5.3. Visualizing influencers

While symptoms typically represent "what" people are feeling, influencers represent "why" people are feeling certain ways. What we have done so far is to bring a structure to the "why" part of mental well-being so that we can categorically and quantitatively analyze the risk and protective factors that affect mental well-being.

There are a total of twelve influencers: positives and negatives of ESI, ISI, EPI, IPI, EMI, and IMI. These twelve influencers are categorical variables that constitute the risk and protective factors. With the defined structure, it is now possible to keep track of influencers over time and visualize the trend. For example, one can pick the most influential positive and negative factors of the day and mark it on a notebook or calendar, like "Positive ESI, Negative ISI." In this case, the most influential positive factor of the day was ESI, external social influencer, like something good or fun on a social side. The most influential negative factor of the day was ISI, the internal social influencer, like low esteem or lack of confidence. If you keep a record like this on a daily basis, and tally up after a period of time, one can create a graph to visualize the trend. The figure below is an example of such trend as a distribution of twelve influencers recorded over time.

(Note to readers: To make this graph, I used a special software tool that collects the influencer data and displays a graph. If you are interested, you can download the software from a mobile app store with a search keyword "Mood Cow Dashboard." It's free and available on both iOS and Android phones and tablets.)

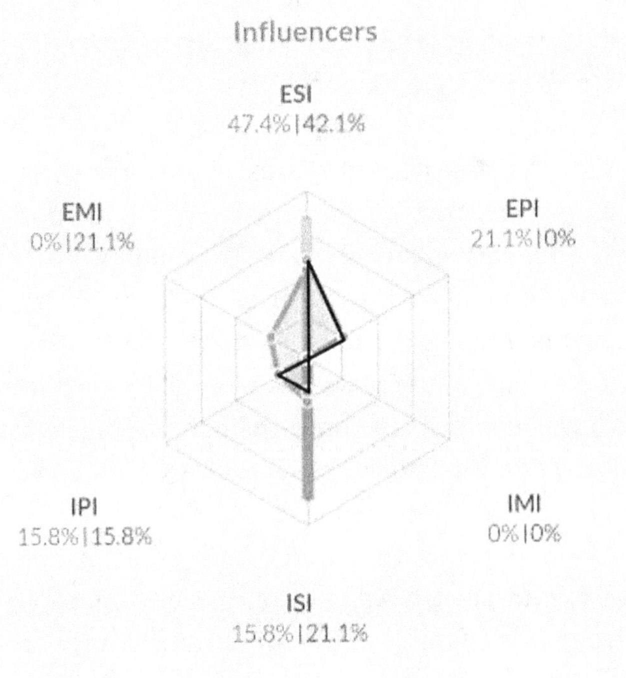

Figure 20. Influencer diagram

The six categorical dimensions are visualized as a hexagonal radar chart. The positive influencers are marked with color green (or dark lines in black and white prints); the negative with color red (or gray lines in black and white prints). The solid green and red bars (gray and dark lines, respectively) are the last entry data. In the figure, the last data of positive influencer was ESI and the last entry on negative influencer was ISI.

The green area (dark line area) in the radar chart shows the distribution of positive influencers, reflecting the percentage of occurrence for each influencer type. The numerical value is noted in each dimension in color green (or on the left side in black and white prints). For example, on ESI (at the top of the hexagonal graph), the number on the left shows 47.4%. It means that the positive ESI was 47.4% of all the positive influencers that have been marked during the period. So, one can say that almost half of this person's protective factor is external social.

Similarly, the red area (light gray area) in the radar chart shows the distribution of negative influencers, reflecting the percentage of occurrence for each influencer type. The numerical value is noted in each dimension in color red. For example, on ESI (at the top of the hexagonal graph), the number on the right shows 42.1%. It means that the negative ESI was 42.1% of all the negative influencers that have been marked during the period. So, one can say that the majority of this person's risk factor is external social.

It is common to have external social influencers as the dominant factors for both positive and negative. Many people suffer from stress from work, family, and relationships. These are external social influencers. But many of the same people find comforts in social events and experiences like hanging out with friends and family. These are also external social influencers.

How to read the influencer diagram

Simply put, you look at the shape of red (or the area of light gray lines) to recognize what's hurting the individual. You look at the shape of green (or the area of dark lines) to recognize what's helping the individual.

By color and shape, the influencer diagram indicates the tendency of risk and protective factors over a period of time. A large value implies that the associated influencer type is influential to the individual. A small value implies less influence.

For example, in case of the figure, the red's largest is ESI (42.1%), followed by EMI and ISI (both 21.1%) and IPI (15.8%). This indicates that the individual is suffering mostly from the external social stress, with some negative factors coming from external mental (bullying), internal social (negative attitude, low self-esteem), and internal physical (illness).

On the positive side, the largest value is at ESI (47.4%), followed by EPI (21.1%), IPI and ISI (both 15.8%). This indicates that the comfort is coming from mostly external social factor (friends, family), with some others from external physical (exercise, food, music, weather), internal physical (good health), and internal social (positive attitude).

As illustrated in this example, by capturing the influencers for a period of time, one can construct a personalized profile of risk and protective factors. This quantitative profile allows statistical analysis and visualization at an individual level and also at a population level. I conducted a field study to empirically prove the utility and effectiveness of the method.

5.4. Empirical study

To determine the practicality of the influencer method, a field study with one hundred participants was conducted. The study was designed to answer two questions.

Can the system identify risk and protective factors for mental well-being?

Can the general public understand and use the method?

These two questions address utility and usability, respectively, of the influencer method, and consequently prove its practicality. If the method works for the general public, and people can use it, then by definition, it is practical.

Method

One hundred factory workers in northern Japan were asked to record their mood, negative influencers, and positive influencers every day for 20 days from April 25 to May 14, 2016. The workers were mostly high school graduates but some with college degrees. Each participant was given a score sheet to record data at home (see sample below).

	Date	Time	Mood	Negative influencer	Positive influencer
	月日	時分	★気分★	▲マイナス要因▲	●プラス要因●
	(mm/dd)	(hh:dd)	(どれか一つに丸印)	(どれか一つに丸印)	(どれか一つに丸印)
1	04/25	21:15	(a) b c d e f	(a) b c d e f	(a) b c d e f
2	04/26	23:00	(a) b c d e f	(a) b c d e f	(a) b c d e f
3	04/27	21:00	a b (c) d e f	(a) b c d e f	(a) b c d e f
4	04/28	3:00	a (b) c d e f	(a) b c d e f	a b (c) d e f
5	04/29	1:00	(a) b c d e f	(a) b c d e f	(a) b c d e f
6	04/30	23:00	(a) b c d e f	(a) b c d e f	(a) b c d e f
7	05/01	20:15	(a) b c d e f	a b c (d) e f	a b (c) d e f
8	05/02	20:45	(a) b c d e f	(a) b c d e f	(a) b c d e f
9	05/03	22:45	(a) b c d e f	a b c (d) e f	a b (c) d e f
10	05/04	21:00	(a) b c d e f	a b c (d) e f	a b (c) d e f
11	05/05	21:45	(a) b c d e f	a b c (d) e f	a b (c) d e f
12	05/06	21:20	(a) b c d e f	(a) b c d e f	(a) b c d e f
13	05/07	22:00	(a) b c d e f	a b (c) d e f	a b (c) d e f
14	05/08	23:00	(a) b c d e f	a b c (d) e f	(a) b c d e f
15	05/09	23:00	a b (c) d e f	(a) b c d e f	(a) b c d e f
16	05/10	22:00	a b (c) d e f	(a) b c d e f	(a) b c d e f
17	05/11	21:00	a b (c) d e f	(a) b c d e f	(a) b c d e f
18	05/12	24:00	a (b) c d e f	(a) b c d e f	a b (c) d e f
19	05/13	23:00	(a) b c d e f	(a) b c d e f	(a) b c d e f
20	05/14	21:00	(a) b c d e f	a b c (d) e f	a b (c) d e f

Figure 21. Sample score sheet used in the field study

On the score sheet, participants were asked to write down the time of record, and mark one of six choices for mood, negative influencers, and positive influencers. No training or explanation about the selections of mood and influencers was given, except a few descriptive keywords on the score sheet as shown below.

Mood:

a. *Fine / Happy,*

b. *Tired,*

c. *Anxious,*

d. *Sad,*

e. *Agitated / Angry,*

f. *Depressed.*

Negative influencers:

a. *(ESI) Stress from work, school, family, friends (exclude bullying), financial problems, accidents, other social events and circumstances.*

b. *ISI) Low self-esteem, negative personality (pessimism, perfectionism).*

c. *(EPI) Medications, alcohol, domestic violence, bad weather.*

d. *(IPI) Poor physical health (illness, injury, lack of sleep, exhaustion).*

e. *(EMI) Bullying at work, school, home, neighborhood.*

f. *(IMI) Symptoms of mental disorder.*

Positive influencers:

a.   *(ESI) Work, family, friends, performance, festivals and events.*

b.   *(ISI) Good self-esteem, positive personality, motivation, strong will.*

c.   *(EPI) Activities, food, medication, music, hobby, exercise, travel, good weather.*

d.   *(IPI) Good physical health.*

e.   *(EMI) Goodwill by someone, charity, spiritual activities.*

f.   *(IMI) Faith, Praying.*

Also on the score sheet, the participants were asked to mark their gender, age group, and a multiple choice answer to the following question: *"Did you understand the meaning of negative and positive influencers?"*

Participation was voluntary, and no incentive or reward was given to the participants. No feedback or visual aid (e.g. graphs) was provided to the participants. After the 20-day period, all one hundred score sheets were retrieved.

Key findings 1

The majority of participants (65%) understood the meaning of negative and positive influencers for their mental well-being.

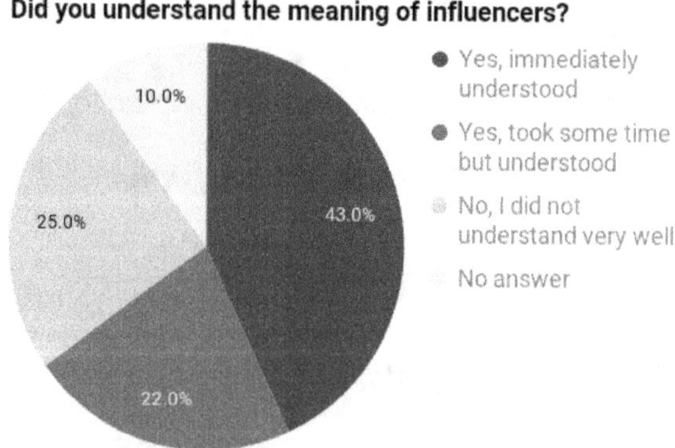

Figure 22. Participant response to user question

To the question of "Did you understand the meaning of negative and positive influencers?", 43% of the participants responded "Yes, immediately understood." 22% responded "Yes, took some time but understood." 25% responded "No, I did not understand very well." 10% did not answer the question.

Lack of clarification about the terms "positive" and "negative" may have confused people who responded that they did not understand very well. On the score sheets, some participants marked positive influencers, but no negatives when they were feeling fine, and marked negative influencers but no positives when they were not feeling fine. Better use of terms and explanations may have avoided their confusion.

Considering the fact that all one hundred score sheets were completed, albeit some blank spots, and the fact that the study did not provide any detailed explanation of the influencers, the results provided a strong evidence that the general public can understand and use the influencer method.

Key findings 2

Risk and protective factors were identified for individuals and the entire group. During the 20-day period, 76 out of 100 participants (76%) marked "Tired" at least once, 46 people (46%) marked "Sad", 45 people (45%) marked "Anxious", 26 people (26%) marked "Angry", and 13 people (13%) marked "Depressed."

What are the factors that make them feel in certain ways, and how are they coping with them? They are important questions from a public health perspective.

How is a specific individual feeling, what is affecting this person, how is this person coping with it, and does this person need help?

If so, how? They are important questions from a clinical practice perspective.

These questions can only be answered if there is a tool that can identify risk and protective factors at an individual level and a population level. The field study data show that the influencer method is capable.

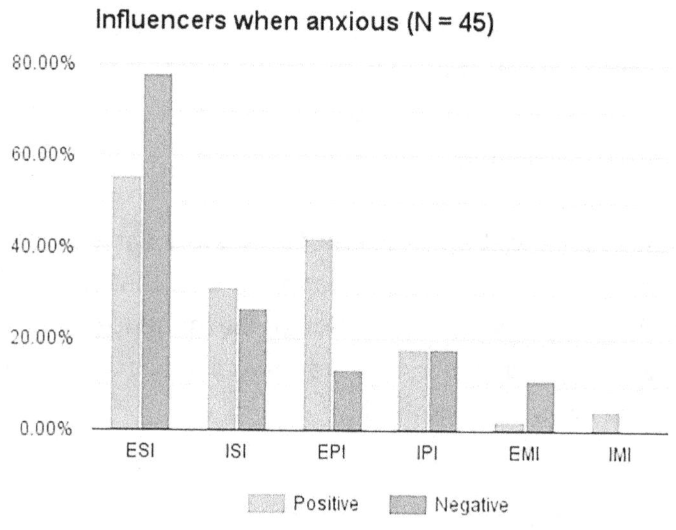

Figure 23. Influencers when feeling anxious (population view)

Forty five out of 100 participants (45%) noted that they felt anxious at least once during the 20-day period. Figure 23 shows the percentage of people who selected particular influencers when feeling "Anxious." The figure depicts the consolidated profile of the risk and protective factors for this group.

Social stress is by far the number one factor for their anxiety (Negative ESI 78%), followed by ISI 27% and IPI 18%. Having EMI at 11% means that five people are experiencing anxiety because of bullying. Another external influencer EPI is at 13%, meaning that six people are experiencing anxiety because of some external physical elements, potentially drugs or domestic violence.

Positive influencers are more spread. The top two, ESI 56% and EPI 42% indicate that the majority rely on social and physical factors to cope with their anxiety. However, ISI at 31% means that almost one third of the group rely on their personal will and strength for coping. In other words, they are "toughing it out" alone. Many mental health experts, especially suicide specialists, know that relying on self-will without seeking outside help is not a good coping approach.

Figure 24 through 28 show the consolidated profiles of the risk and protective factors for other mood types.

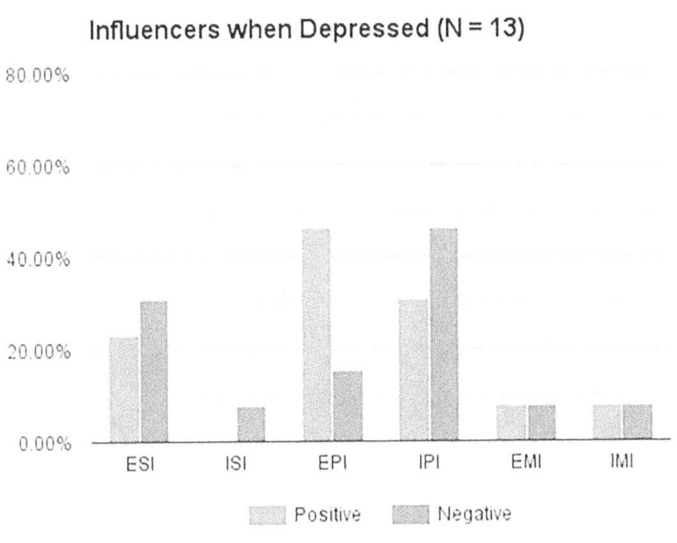

Figure 24. Influencers chosen when feeling depressed (population view)

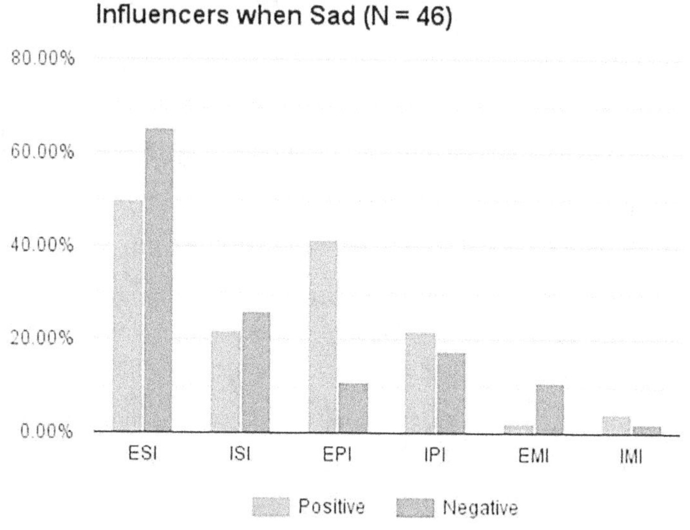

Figure 25. Influencers chosen when feeling sad (population view)

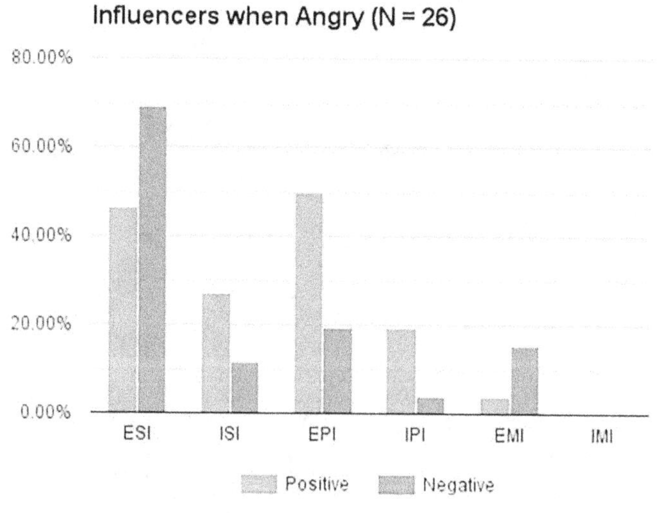

Figure 26. Influencers chosen when feeling angry (population view)

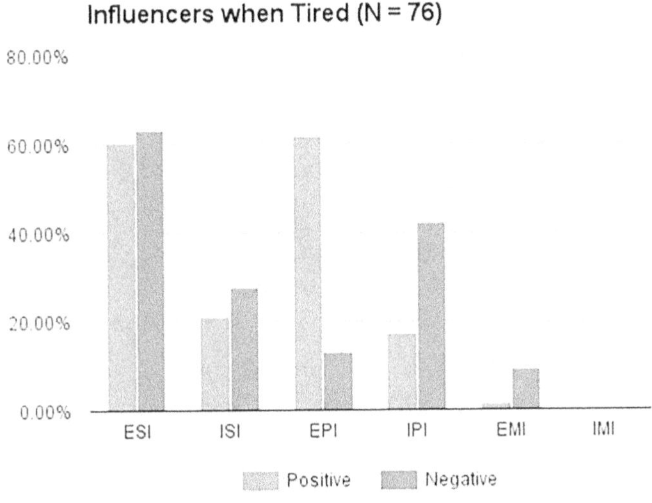

Figure 27. Influencers chosen when feeling tired (population view)

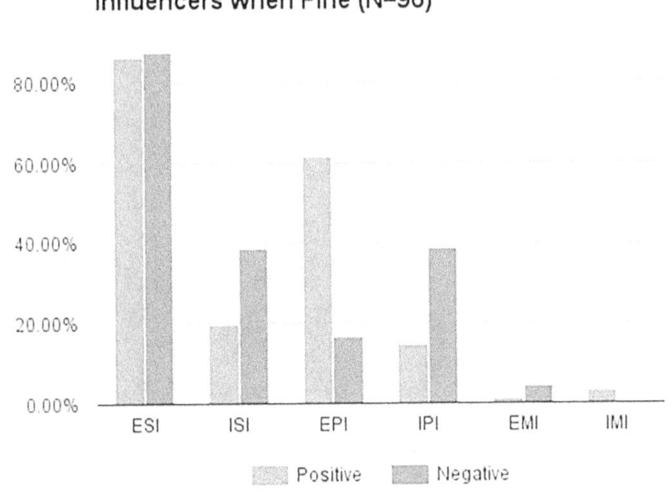

Figure 28. Influencers chosen when feeling fine (population view)

While the above analysis provides insights at a population level, what about an individual level?

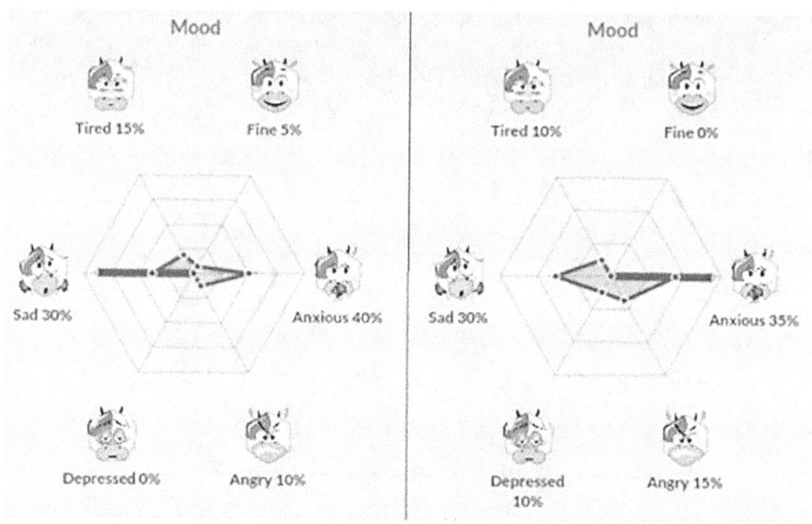

Figure 29. Mood distribution of two individuals (Data#051, #052)

Figure 29 shows two individuals' mood distribution over the 20-day period. Notice that they appear very similar. They both felt anxious (40% & 35%), sad (both 30%), angry (10% & 15%), tired (15% & 10%), and fine (5% & 0%) at an almost identical rate. Without knowing their risk and protective factors, we would falsely assume that they need similar intervention support.

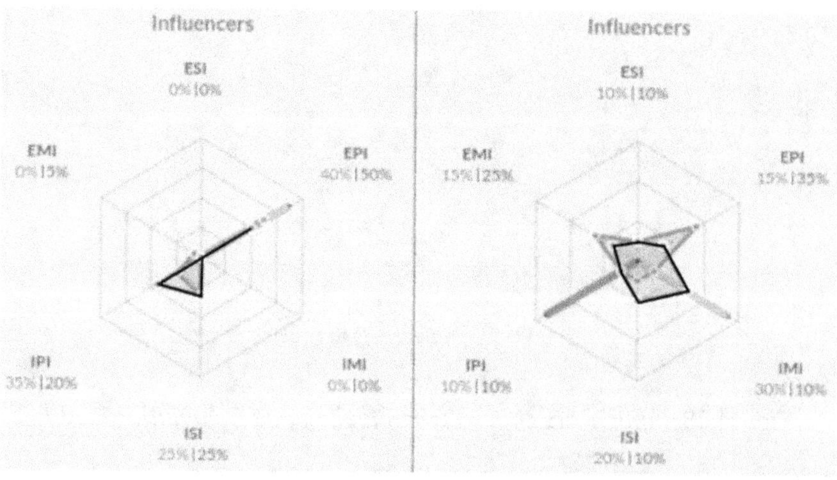

Figure 30. Influencer distribution of two individuals (Data#051, #052)

Figure 30 shows their influencer distributions. Notice how different their influencers are, even though their mood distributions looked similar in Figure 29. The left side (Data#051) has high negative EPI (50%), and moderate ISI (25%) and IPI (20%), shown in light gray. This individual is not suffering from social stress but suffering from external and internal physical elements. This individual's positive influencers are EPI (40%), IPI (35%), and ISI (25%), shown in dark gray lines.

The right side (Data#052) on the other hand has more spread profile with negative EPI (35%), negative EMI (25%), and the rest at 10% each, shown in light gray lines. Negative EMI 25% indicates a moderate influence of bullying. This individual's positive influencers are also spread with positive IMI (30%), ISI (20%), and the rest at 10 to 15% each, shown in dark gray lines. Positive IMI means faith and spiritual, and positive ISI means self-will, indicate strong reliance on self-help.

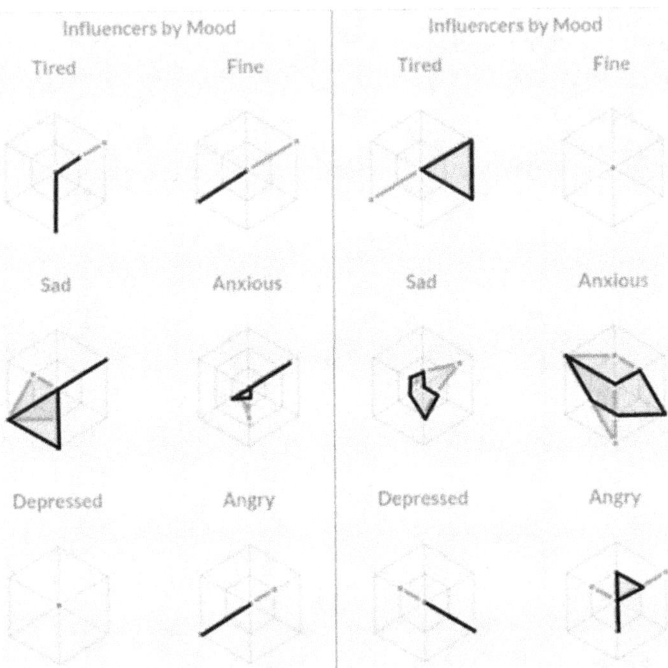

Figure 31. Influencer choice by mood types (Data#051, #052)

Figure 31 shows the two individuals' influencers by mood types. Notice how different they are between the two individuals. For example, when feeling anxious, the person on the left marked EPI and ISI only (shown in light gray lines), indicating that anxiety comes from physical elements and low self-esteem. The person is relying mostly on physical elements to cope with anxiety (shown in dark gray lines).

The person on right suffers from multiple influencers, most notably negative EMI (shown in light gray lines), indicating bullying is causing anxiety. The positive influencers are EMI and IMI (shown in dark gray lines), indicating that the person is relying on spiritual experience and goodwill to cope with anxiety.

Conclusion

The field study confirmed the affirmative answers to both questions and provided empirical evidence that the influencer method can be a practical mental care monitoring tool.

CHAPTER 6

EARLY CHILDHOOD MENTAL CARE

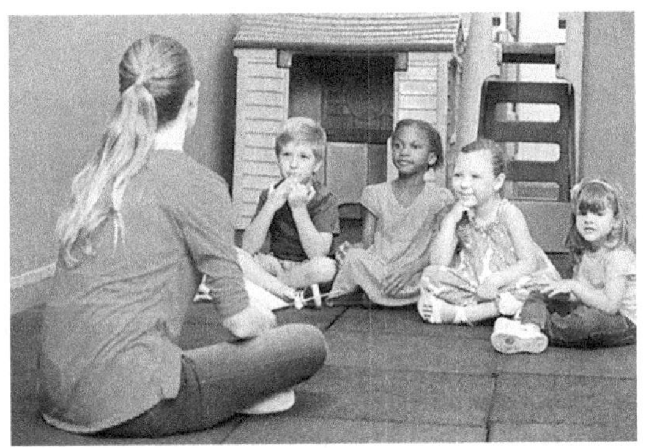

6.1. Introduction

The right age to build mental resilience

FOUR MILLION BABIES are born each year in the US. By the time they reach the age of three, they develop sufficient cognitive and motor skills to recognize, express, and verbalize feelings of self and others. By age five, most of them enter standardized school systems with more emphasis on academic performance than health education.

In the US, National Health Education Standards (NHES)[42] establish curriculum standards to promote healthy behaviors for all students from pre-kindergarten to grade 12. In NHES, there is a special module for mental and emotional health (MEH). While most states adopt and endorse NHES, many do not mandate the MEH module in their public schools. As a result, many students in K-12 do not learn mental and emotional health at school. This situation is likely to continue because of the financial constraints in public education, and the primary focus on academic achievement.

It seems therefore important to prepare young children with mental care before they enter a school system. The narrow window of three years between the age of three and five is a golden opportunity to build their social and mental resilience and the foundation of mental care.

Lack of preparedness in health care

In the US, most children between the age of three and five see their pediatricians at least once a year for well-child visits.[43] This is a time for parents and physicians to go over children's physiological and behavioral development, including medical history, measurement, sensory screening, immunizations, dental referral, anticipatory guidance, and developmental and behavioral assessment.[44] Parents are looking for well-child visits to receive guidance from pediatricians on the social and emotional development of their young children. However, according to research,[45] many parents feel that they are not getting enough information from pediatricians on behavioral topics such as discipline and learning.

According to research,[46] almost 90% of pediatricians are not confident in their training or ability to manage children's behavioral and emotional problems. The reasons are lack of time, liabilities, lack of available mental health providers to refer children, and long waits for children to be seen by mental-health providers. The increasing number of mandates in pediatric practice guidelines, coupled with increasing pressure on reimbursement income, is restricting their time spent with patients.

In the meantime, the demand is high for health-care intervention for children's behavioral and emotional problems. According to research,[46] 20% of children in the US have a behavioral or emotional disorder, and one third of children will have a behavioral or emotional disorder diagnosed by 16 years of age.

Because of the lack of preparedness in health care, parents must look somewhere else for guidance for their children's emotional and behavioral development.

6.2. Early childhood education

The current trend in early childhood education is a head start in STEM: science, technology, engineering, and math. This movement is pushed by technology and education companies, capitalizing on young parents' desire for their children's future success. On the other hand, a number of research organizations are advocating for social and emotional development over academic skills for young children. These organizations are funded by the government, most notably the US Department of Education and the US Department of Health and Human Services. In other words, commercial interests are pushing STEM, while government studies are calling for mental care for young children.

The Pyramid Model

The most well-known program for social and emotional development for young children is the Pyramid Model.[47] It was developed by the Center for the Social and Emotional Foundations for Early Learning (CSEFEL) at Vanderbilt University[48] and the Technical

Assistance Center on Social Emotional Intervention for Youth Children (TACSEI) at the University of South Florida.[49] Both of these institutions are funded by the US government to disseminate research and evidence-based practices to early childhood programs across the country, and developed training materials, videos, and print resources for families and preschools.

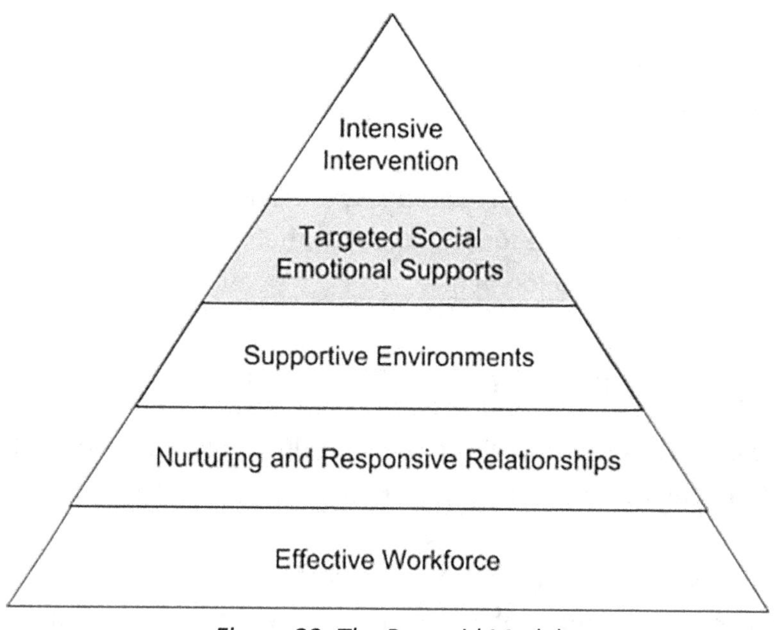

Figure 32. The Pyramid Model

The model is called "pyramid" because of its tiered structure that represents the stacked foundations to support children's social emotional development. At the base is the trained workforce providing the effective care. Building on the workforce base is nurturing and responsive relationships with children, families and care-providers. Building on the relationships is supportive environments, where children can learn appropriate behavior through safe, nurturing, hands-on, stimulating activities. Building on the environments is the curricula for social emotional supports, specifically designed to address early signs of challenging behavior.

Finally, the top tier is intensive intervention for children who need special help.

The three base tiers of workforce, relationships, and environments are the core of general early childhood education, and relate to the promotion of preventive mental care. At the top tier of intensive intervention is the special program in education, and relates to indicated prevention and corrective treatment. Of the five tiers in the Pyramid Model, the second tier of targeted social emotional supports is the most relevant to universal prevention with specific curricula. The curricula promote the following social emotional skills:

- Confidence
- Capacity to develop relationships with peers and adults
- Concentration and persistence when facing challenging tasks
- Ability to effectively communicate emotions
- Ability to listen to instructions and be attentive
- Ability to solve social problems

CSEFEL and TACSEI have developed training materials for families and preschools to teach the skills to children. The materials are available from the following websites.

CSEFEL: http://csefel.vanderbilt.edu/

TACSEI: (NCPMI):http://challengingbehavior.cbcs.usf.edu/index.html

National Health Education Standards

While the Pyramid Model was designed for families, caregivers, and preschools, the National Health Education Standards (NHES) are designed for teachers, administrators, and policymakers in designing or selecting curricula, allocating instructional resources, and assessing achievement and progress for students from pre-Kindergarten to grade 12.[42] The NHES were created by the Joint Committee on National Health Education Standards with members from American Public Health Association, American School Health Association, and the Society of Health and Physical Educators. The NHES became the accepted standards for health education by most states in the US.

- **Standard 1:** Students will comprehend concepts related to health promotion and disease prevention to enhance health.

- **Standard 2:** Students will analyze the influence of family, peers, culture, media, technology, and other factors on health behaviors.

- **Standard 3:** Students will demonstrate the ability to access valid information, products, and services to enhance health.

- **Standard 4:** Students will demonstrate the ability to use interpersonal communication skills to enhance health and avoid or reduce health risks.

- **Standard 5:** Students will demonstrate the ability to use decision-making skills to enhance health.

- **Standard 6:** Students will demonstrate the ability to use goal-setting skills to enhance health.

- **Standard 7:** Students will demonstrate the ability to practice health-enhancing behaviors and avoid or reduce health risks.

- **Standard 8:** Students will demonstrate the ability to advocate for personal, family, and community health.

Health Education Curriculum Analysis Tool (HECAT)

HECAT[50] provides a guideline to help schools and school districts conduct a clear, complete, and consistent analysis of health education curricula based on the National Health Education Standards. There are nine modules:

- **Module 1:** Alcohol and other drugs

- **Module 2:** Healthy eating

- **Module 3:** <u>Mental and emotional health</u>

- **Module 4:** Personal health and wellness

- **Module 5:** Physical activity

- **Module 6:** Safety

- **Module 7:** Tobacco

- **Module 8:** Violence Prevention

- **Module 9:** Comprehensive health education

In the Module 3 on mental and emotional health curriculum, healthy behavior objectives (HBO) are defined as follows:

- **HBO 1:** Express feelings in a healthy way.

- **HBO 2:** Engage in activities that are mentally and emotionally healthy.

- **HBO 3:** Prevent and manage interpersonal conflict in healthy ways.

- **HBO 4:** Prevent and manage emotional stress and anxiety in healthy ways.

- **HBO 5:** Use self-control and impulse-control strategies to promote health.

- **HBO 6:** Get help for troublesome thoughts, feelings, or actions for oneself and others.

- **HBO 7:** Show tolerance and acceptance of differences in others.

- **HBO 8:** Establish and maintain healthy relationships.

Mental and Emotional Health (MEH) Education Standards for pre-K to Grade 2

Based on the NHES and HECAT, specific MEH education standards for pre-K to Grade 2 are defined.

Standard 1: Concept comprehension

- **MEH 1.2.1:** Explain the importance of talking with parents and other trusted adults about feelings.

- **MEH 1.2.2:** Identify appropriate ways to express and deal with feelings.

- **MEH 1.2.3:** Explain the relationship between feelings and behavior.

- **MEH 1.2.4:** Describe the difference between bullying and teasing.

- **MEH 1.2.5:** Explain the importance of respecting the personal space and boundaries of others.

- **MEH 1.2.6:** Explain why it is wrong to tease or bully others.

- **MEH 1.2.7:** Identify the benefits of healthy family relationships.

- **MEH 1.2.8:** Identify the benefits of healthy peer relationships.

Standard 2: Analysis of external influence

- **MEH 2.2.1:** Identify relevant influences of family on mental and emotional health practices and behaviors.

- **MEH 2.2.2:** Identify relevant influences of school on mental and emotional health practices and behaviors.

- **MEH 2.2.3:** Identify relevant influences of media and technology on mental and emotional health practices and behaviors.

- **MEH 2.2.4:** Describe positive influences of mental and emotional health practices and behaviors.

- **MEH 2.2.5:** Describe negative influences of mental and emotional health practices and behaviors.

Standard 3: Demonstration of resource access

- **MEH 3.2.1:** Identify trusted adults at home who can help promote mental and emotional health.

- **MEH 3.2.2:** Identify trusted adults and professionals in school who can help promote mental and emotional health (e.g. school nurse, school counselor).

- **MEH 3.2.3:** Identify trusted adults and professionals in the community who can help promote mental and emotional health (e.g. counselors, social workers, healthcare providers).

- **MEH 3.2.4:** Explain how to locate school health helpers who can help with mental and emotional health (e.g. school nurse, school counselor).

- **MEH 3.2.5:** Explain how to locate community health helpers who can help with mental and emotional health (e.g. counselors, healthcare providers).

- **MEH 3.2.6:** Demonstrate how to locate school health helpers to enhance mental and emotional health.

Standard 4: Demonstration of communication skills

- **MEH 4.2.1:** Demonstrate how to effectively communicate needs, wants, and feelings in healthy ways.

- **MEH 4.2.2:** Demonstrate effective active listening skills including paying attention, and verbal and nonverbal feedback.

- **MEH 4.2.3:** Demonstrate effective refusal skills to avoid participating in emotionally unhealthy behaviors.

- **MEH 4.2.4:** Demonstrate how to effectively tell a trusted adult when feeling threatened or harmed.

- **MEH 4.2.5:** Describe how to effectively communicate care and concern for others.

Standard 5: Demonstration of decision-making skills

- **MEH 5.2.1:** Identify situations which need a decision related to mental and emotional health (e.g. dealing with interpersonal conflict, managing anger).

- **MEH 5.2.2:** Describe how family, peers or media influence a decision related to mental and emotional health.

- **MEH 5.2.3:** Explain the potential positive and negative outcomes from decisions related to mental and emotional health (e.g. dealing with interpersonal conflict, managing anger).

- **MEH 5.2.4:** Describe when help is needed and when it is not needed to make a mentally and emotionally healthy decision (e.g. dealing with interpersonal conflict, managing anger).

Standard 6: Demonstration of goal-seeking skills

- **MEH 6.2.1:** Identify a realistic personal short-term goal to improve or maintain positive mental and emotional health.

- **MEH 6.2.2:** Take steps to achieve the goal to improve or maintain positive mental and emotional health.

- **MEH 6.2.3:** Identify people who can help achieve a goal to improve or maintain positive mental and emotional health.

Standard 7: Demonstration of healthy behaviors

- **MEH 7.2.1:** Identify mental and emotional health practices that reduce or prevent health risks.

- **MEH 7.2.2:** Demonstrate healthy mental and emotional health practices.

- **MEH 7.2.3:** Make a commitment to practice healthy mental and emotional health behaviors.

Standard 8: Demonstration of health promotion

- **MEH 8.2.1:** Make requests to others to promote personal mental and emotional health practices.

- **MEH 8.2.2:** Demonstrate how to encourage peers to make healthy mental and emotional health choices.

Even though well structured, most states do not mandate the MEH curriculum in their public schools, and as a result, students in K-12 do not learn mental and emotional health.

6.3. Early childhood mental care curriculum at home

We learned so far that the NHES provides well-defined learning objectives and curriculum structure for young children's mental and emotional health, though they are not utilized much in public schools in the US. We also learned that the Pyramid Model provides well-researched curricula and training materials for teachers and families. As the NHES and Pyramid Model share the same goal, their resources are synergistic. But since they are designed primarily for schools, teachers, and trained caregivers, the curricula seem overwhelming and difficult to use at home by typical parents.

Here I propose a simplified curriculum that can be used at home by parents with children between the age of three and five. While the main structure is derived from the NHES and Pyramid Model, the learning objectives are narrowed down to three core skills based on the mental care principles.

The goal of the curriculum is to build mental resilience in children. To achieve the goal, the curriculum helps children and their family members acquire basic skills to prevent and manage emotional stress in healthy ways. Specifically, the curriculum teaches three core skills:

- Ability to recognize and verbalize emotion,
- Ability to recognize influencers, and
- Ability to self-calm and communicate for help.

Skill 1 - Ability to recognize and verbalize emotion

Children at age three can express a range of emotions such as being happy, sad, mad, or bored.[51] Their vocabulary is rapidly growing with 200 or more words, and they can string together three- or four-word sentences.[52] This is an opportune moment to teach them to apply their verbal skills to express their feelings in words.

Putting feelings into words has long been known to help manage negative emotional experiences but the exact mechanism was not known until recently. With advancement in neuroimaging techniques, scientists identified a neural pathway of diminished response to negative experiences when feelings are verbalized.[53] In other words, when we verbalize our negative feelings, like anger and sadness, our brains show reduced response, and the degree of negative feeling is lessened. This mechanism is called affective labeling, and it's been the underlying principle of psychotherapies. Now that the scientists have discovered the evidence of affective labeling in brain imaging, we should encourage children to name their negative feeling instead of keeping it to themselves.

The ability to recognize and verbalize feelings is an important social skill for young children. It gives them a healthier way to express themselves than resorting to poor behavior that often arises from emotional stress. It also promotes a constructive social environment through communication with others. And as evidenced in neuroscience, putting feelings into words reduces the effect of stressors.

Skill 2 - Ability to recognize influencers

While the first skill enables children to recognize "what" they are feeling, the second skill enables them to recognize "why" they are feeling certain ways. Developmental science of early childhood provides evidence of child-parent communication about influencers, not the feeling itself, as the key factor for children's mental and behavioral development. Recent studies emphasize the importance of "why" in promoting a healthy relationship. The process is referred to as "mentalizing."[54]

In addition to recognizing negative influencers, children need to learn to recognize positive influencers that help them overcome the stress and effect of negative influencers. Positive influencers for young children typically revolve around external social and physical elements such as being close to moms, dads, pets, familiar toys, games and favorite food. For example, if a child is feeling upset at a playground, he could first voice to himself "I'm feeling mad", and then he could think of his mom's face and remembers that he can go home soon to see her. In this way, using a cognitive mode of mental care, children can learn to identify, recognize, and use influencers to regulate their behavior. It's easier to control how you behave than how you feel.

Like balancing a teeter-totter, knowing what helps them feel, think, and behave better in the presence of stress builds resilience in children. This matches perfectly with what the World Health Organization advocates: "preventive interventions work by focusing on reducing risk factors and enhancing protective factors associated with mental ill-health."[55]

Skill 3 - Ability to self-calm and communicate for help

The ability to understand social rules and manners gives confidence for children to express their feelings properly and communicate with adults for help. To do so in real situations, children must also know how to calm themselves first before they communicate. The easiest and most effective self-calm skill for young children is deep breathing. Exhale slowly for 5 seconds, then inhale for 5 seconds, and repeat 3 times. This 30-second time out is all it takes.

Recent studies provide an evidence of controlled breathing as an effective self-calming technique.[56] Here is how and why deep breathing is effective. People typically breathe 12 to 20 times a minute at rest. When stressed, people experience fast heart rate and shallow breathing. The diaphragm's range of motion is limited with shallow breathing, resulting in less than fully oxygenated air. Slow, deep breathing encourages full oxygen exchange, improving the chemical balance of the body. Deep breathing also activates the nerve system and improves the balance between sympathetic and parasympathetic nervous systems, driving heart rate down and lowering blood pressure. Deep breathing has been utilized as a major component of relaxation techniques for stress management, such as yoga and meditation for years.

Curriculum structure

In the proposed curriculum, eight NHES standards are condensed to three topics with five lessons each.

Topic 1: How you feel (NHES Standard 1)

Topic 2: Why do you feel certain ways (NHES Standard 2)

Topic 3: How to self-calm and communicate (NHES Standards 3, 4, 5, 6, 7, 8)

Each lesson should take less than an hour per day. Each lesson consists of images, stories, activities, and assessments. Repeat all three topics in cycles for reinforcement.

Early childhood mental care curriculum

(Week 1) Topic 1 - How you feel

Objectives: Children learn to:

- Identify appropriate ways to express and deal with feelings (MEH 1.2.2).

- Explain the relationship between feelings and behavior (MEH 1.2.3).

- Explain the importance of respecting the personal space and boundaries of others (MEH 1.2.5).

- Explain why it is wrong to tease or bully others (MEH 1.2.6).

Lessons:

- (Monday) Lesson 1: Different types of feelings

- (Tuesday) Lesson 2: Feelings and behaviors

- (Wednesday) Lesson 3: Good ways and bad ways to express feelings

- (Thursday) Lesson 4: Feelings of other people

- (Friday) Lesson 5: Teasing and bullying

(Week 2) Topic 2 - Why do you feel certain ways

Objectives: Children learn to:

- Identify positive influences on feelings and behaviors (MEH 2.2.1, 2.2.2, 2.2.3, 2.2.4).

- Identify negative influences on feelings and behaviors (MEH 2.2.1, 2.2.2, 2.2.3, 2.2.5).

Lessons:

- (Monday) Lesson 6: Influencers in family and school

- (Tuesday) Lesson 7: Influencers in TV, movies, music, video games

- (Wednesday) Lesson 8: Influence by weather, food, outdoor activities

- (Thursday) Lesson 9: Influence by injury and illness

- (Friday) Lesson 10: Other influencers

(Week 3) Topic 3 - How to self-calm and communicate

Objectives: Children learn to:

- Identify trusted adults at home and professionals in school and in community who can help promote emotional health (MEH 3.2.1, 3.2.2, 3.3.3).

- Demonstrate how to effectively communicate needs, wants, and feelings in healthy ways (MEH 4.2.1, 4.2.2, 4.2.3, 4.2.4, 4.2.5).

- Identify situations which need a decision related to emotional health (MEH 5.2.1).

- Demonstrate healthy emotional health practices (MEH 6.2.2, MEH 7.2.2).

- Demonstrate how to encourage peers to make healthy emotional health choices (MEH 8.2.2).

Lessons:

- (Monday) Lesson 11: Self-help and self-calming

- (Tuesday) Lesson 12: Attention, look, and listen

- (Wednesday) Lesson 13: Help at home, school, and community

- (Thursday) Lesson 14: Needs, wants, feelings

- (Friday) Lesson 15: Healthy choices

In essence, the curriculum's three topics represent the "what," "why," and "how" of feelings. The "what" of feelings teaches children the basics, the "why" builds resilience and promotes healthy relationships, and the "how" provides tools to regulate behavior and make good choices. Suggestions on practical tools and materials for the curriculum are listed in Appendix C.

6.4. Keep it simple

As a concluding section of this chapter, I present a simple, easy routine that anyone, even young children can do to improve and maintain mental wellness. The routine consists of six actions: the sun, hydration / nutrition, exercise, deep breathing, sleep, and goodwill. Plenty of scientific evidence shows that these actions can help you feel, think, and behave better. A printable pamphlet with detailed information is available in Appendix A.

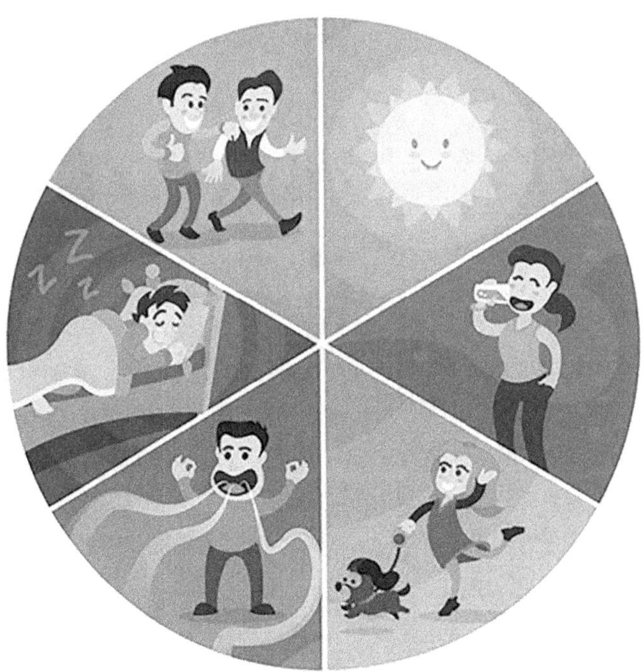

Figure 33. Six actions for better mental well-being

Sunlight - Sunlight is an effective, free, and natural mood enhancer. When you feel a little stressed, anxious, sad, or upset, take a quick break and walk outside or just look out the window.

Hydration / nutrition - Stress can cause dehydration and dehydration can cause stress. Drinking plenty of water can minimize the negative effects of stress on your body and brain. Eat balanced meals and maintain a stable blood sugar level during the day.

Exercise - Even mild forms of exercise can help you relieve stress to fight troubling thoughts. Walk 30 minutes every day, or create your own physical activity plan and stick to it every day.

Deep breathing - Slow, measured breathing is a quick and easy stress reliever, and it can help you cope with negative thoughts better. Try exhaling slowly for 3 to 6 seconds then inhale slowly for 3 to 6 seconds. Repeat this 5 times. Do this whenever you feel a little stressed. It only takes a minute.

Sleep - Good restorative sleep is critical for your body and brain. A balanced diet, hydration, sunlight and exercise can help you fall asleep and stay asleep longer.

Goodwill / social connection - Emotional connection with people and activities can improve your well-being. Give kind, warm, encouraging words and do something nice to your friends, family, colleagues, and even complete strangers. Creative activities can also enhance your well-being. Engage in activities like art, music, dance, drama, writing, poetry, craft works, gardening, cooking, and traveling.

References

42. Centers for Disease Control and Prevention. National Health Education Standards. Retrieved on August 16, 2016 from https://www.cdc.gov/healthyschools/sher/standards/index.htm

43. US National Library of Medicine Medline Plus. *Well-child visits.* Retrieved on April 2018 from https://medlineplus.gov/ency/article/001928.htm

44. Child Trends Databank. *Well-child visits*. October 2014. Retrieved from https://www.childtrends.org/?indicators=well-child-visits

45. Schuster MA, Duan N, Regalado M, Klein DJ. Anticipatory Guidance: What Information Do Parents Receive? What Information Do They Want? *Archives of Pediatrics & Adolescent Medicine.* 2000;154(12):1191–1198. doi:10.1001/archpedi.154.12.1191 https://www.ncbi.nlm.nih.gov/pubmed/11115301

46. Weitzman C, Wegner L. Promoting optimal development: screening for behavioral and emotional problems. *Pediatrics.* American Academy of Pediatrics. 135:384–95. 2015. doi:10.1542/pcds.2014-3716 http://pediatrics.aappublications.org/content/135/2/384

47. The National Center for Pyramid Model Innovations. Pyramid Model Overview. Retrieved from http://challengingbehavior.cbcs.usf.edu/Pyramid/overview/index.html

48. Center on the Social and Emotional Foundations for Early Learning. CSEFEL. Retrieved from http://csefel.vanderbilt.edu/

49. Technical Assistance Center on Social-Emotional Interventions. TACSEI. Retrieved from http://challengingbehavior.cbcs.usf.edu/index.html

50. Centers for Disease Control and Prevention. HECAT: Module MEH Mental and Emotional Health Curriculum. Retrieved from http://www.cdc.gov/healthyyouth/hecat/pdf/hecat_module_meh.pdf

51. Centers for Disease Control and Prevention. Important Milestones: By the End of Three Years (36 Months). Retrieved from https://www.cdc.gov/ncbddd/actearly/milestones/milestones-3yr.html

52. KidsHealth. Communication and Your 2- to 3-Year-Old. Retrieved from http://kidshealth.org/en/parents/comm-2-to-3.html

53. Lieberman, M. D., Eisenberger, N. I., Crockett, M. J., Tom, S. M., Pfeifer, J. H., and Way, B. M. Putting feelings into words: affect labeling disrupts amygdala activity in response to affective stimuli. *Psychological Science*. 18, 421–428. 2007. https://www.ncbi.nlm.nih.gov/pubmed/17576282

54. Gold, C.M. The Developmental Science of Early Childhood: Clinical Applications of Infant Mental Health Concepts from Infancy Through Adolescence. W.W. Norton & Company, 2017. http://books.wwnorton.com/books/The-Developmental-Science-of-Early-Childhood/

55. World Health Organization. Prevention of Mental Disorders: Effective Interventions and Policy Options. Geneva: World Health Organization, 2004. http://www.who.int/mental_health/evidence/en/prevention_of_mental_disorders_sr.pdf

56. LeDoux J.E. Anxious: Using the Brain to Understand and Treat Fear and Anxiety. New York: Viking Penguin. 2015. https://www.penguinrandomhouse.com/books/313935/anxious-by-joseph-ledoux/9780143109044/

SUMMARY OF PART 2

- Established four principles of mental care.

- All feelings are acceptable, but poor behavior is not.

- There are risk and protective factors that influence mental health.

- Mental care is an iterative process.

- Medications and therapies are not the primary tools of mental care; six modes of treatment exist.

- Guided by the first principle, the role of health care and the responsibility of self were defined, and a system tool was created to determine when to seek medical help.

- Guided by the second principle, a process was defined to identify and track risk and protective influencers.

- Guided by the third principle, an iterative self-help process was defined.

- Guided by the principles and national health education standards, an early childhood mental care curriculum was proposed to help parents at home build resilience in children.

Part 3

· · · · · · · · · · · ·

RESOURCE

THE LAST SECTION of this book provides practical resources for self-help. Appendix A provides the six routine actions for mental care. Appendix B provides a list of best first resources for self-help. Appendix C provides lesson materials at home for the early childhood mental care curriculum as outlined in Chapter 6.

Six Routine Actions for Mental Care

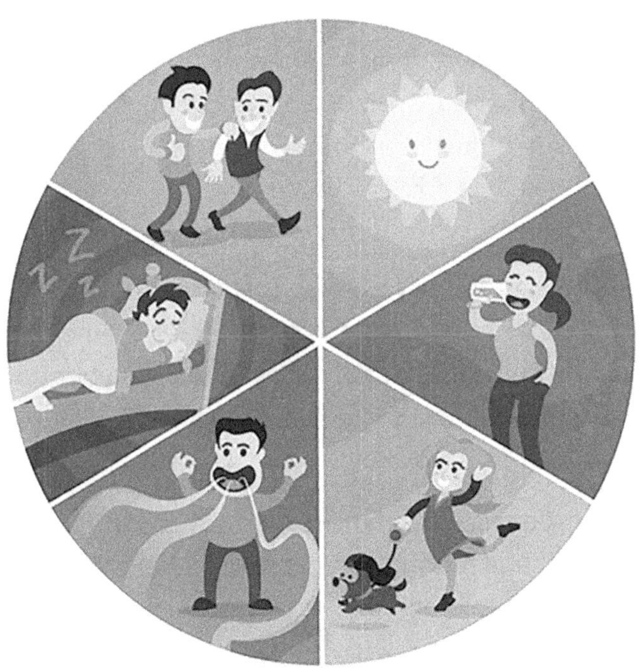

A SIMPLE ROUTINE CAN promote good health, like daily skin and dental care. Mental care is the same. There is plenty of scientific evidence that simple actions can help you feel, think, and behave better. The picture shows six simple actions you can take to improve your mental and emotional well-being every day.

#1 Sun - A sunny day boosts your mood.

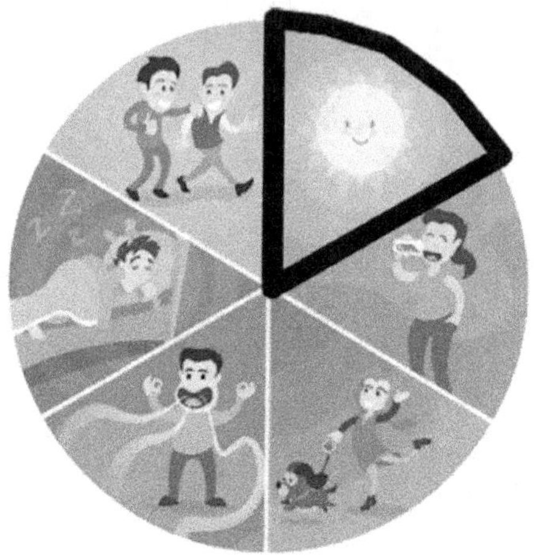

Sunlight is an effective, free, and natural mood enhancer. When you feel a little stressed, anxious, sad, or upset, take a quick break and walk outside or just look out the window. Even sunlight under a cloudy sky may help you feel better.

Why sunlight is good for you? Scientists found that the onset of depression relates to reduced serotonin levels, a type of chemical called a neurotransmitter in the neural system in your body. They found that serotonin levels increase on sunny days more than on darker days.

To learn how scientists found the results, see 57, 58, 59 in the reference section. To find more about the sunlight benefit, these articles are good and easy to read:

- *Unraveling the Sun's Role in Depression* by WebMD: 2002.

- *Benefits of Sunlight: A Bright Spot for Human Health* by M. Nathaniel Mead: 2008.

Caution: Unprotected exposure to UV radiation burns you like a steak. No really — it's a real health risk. Please use appropriate protections like sunglasses and sunblock lotions.

- **Sunlight helps you feel better.**

- **Protect your skin from sunlight.**

- **Make it a routine to keep you healthy.**

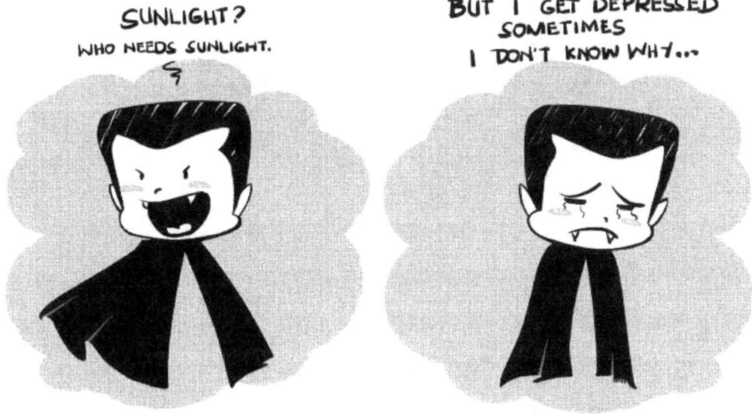

© 2016 Mood Cow

#2 Hydration - Proper hydration and nutrition help balance your mood.

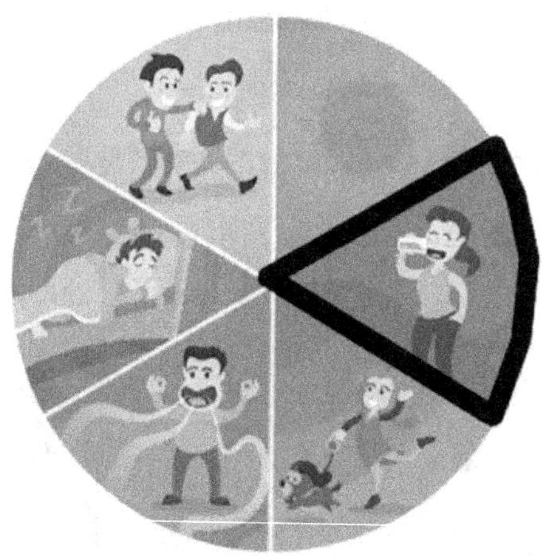

Stress can cause dehydration and dehydration can cause stress. Drinking plenty of water can minimize the negative effects of stress on your body and brain. Check your urine color. If it's pale, good. If it's dark, you need more water. Eat balanced meals and maintain a stable blood sugar level during the day.

Why is hydration good for you? Scientists found that even mild dehydration can affect mood, energy levels, and judgment. They recommend a minimum of 2 liters of water a day (8-ounce glass x 8) to refill the minimal body fluid loss. They also recommend minimizing the consumption of alcohol, caffeine, and sugar. To learn how scientists found the results, see 60, 61, 62 in the reference section. To find more about the hydration benefit, these articles are good and easy to read:

- *Even Mild Dehydration Can Alter Mood* by Colin Poitras: 2012.

- *From bad breath to car accidents, dehydration is a real health threat* by Linda Melone: 2015.

- *Food to Balance Your Mood* by Star Lawrence: 2002.

Caution: Be aware of when to drink and where you'll have to urinate. Ever been caught in traffic and have that urge? Not fun. Drinking an extreme amount of water in a short time can cause water intoxication. Be aware of what you eat. People have different sensitivities to different foods (e.g., gluten).

- **Hydration helps you feel better.**

- **Eat balanced meals.**

- **Make it a routine to keep you healthy.**

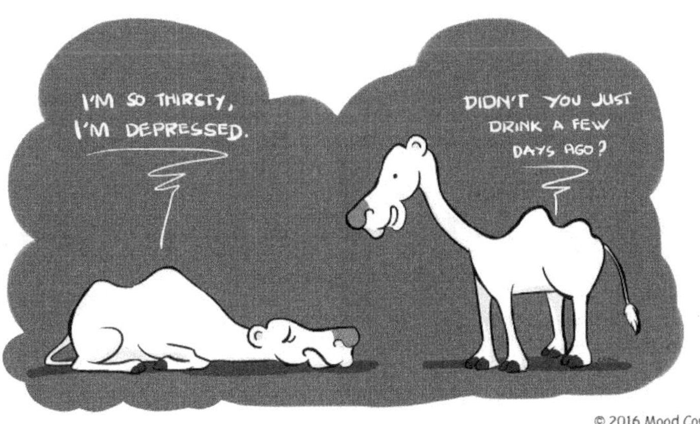

© 2016 Mood Cow

#3 Exercise - Physical activity improves mental well-being.

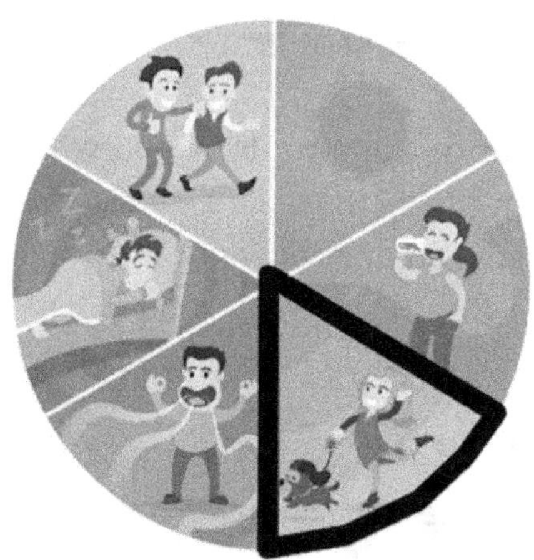

Even mild forms of exercise can help you relieve stress to fight troubling thoughts. Walk 30 minutes every day or create your own physical activity plan and stick to it every day.

Why is exercise good for you? Scientists found that regular participation in moderate-to-vigorous physical activity improves mental well-being and reduces mental health symptoms. To learn how scientists found the results, see 63 in the reference section. To find more about the exercise benefit, these articles are good and easy to read:

- *The Mental Health Benefits of Exercise* by L. Robinson, J. Segal, and M. Smith: 2016.

Caution: If you have a medical problem, check with your doctor before starting a new exercise program to make sure it's safe for you.

- **Exercise helps you feel better.**

- **Make it a routine to keep you healthy.**

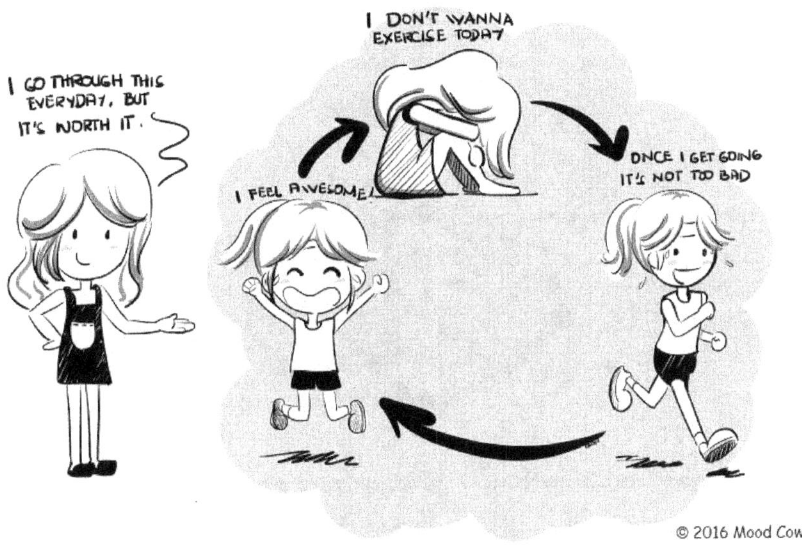

#4 Breathing - Deep abdominal breathing reduces stress.

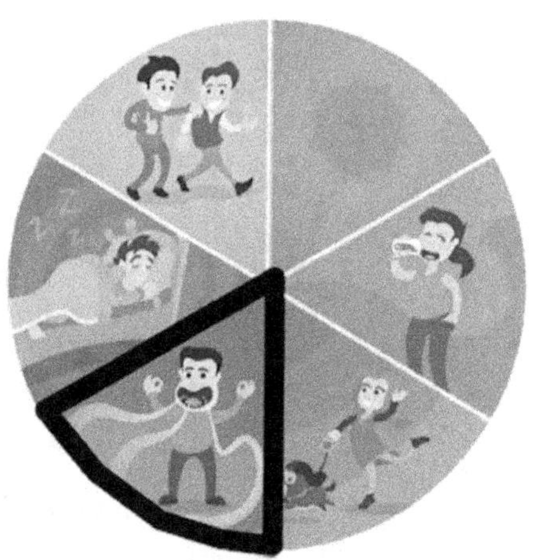

Slow, measured breathing is a quick and easy stress reliever, and it can help you cope with negative thoughts better. Try exhaling slowly for 3 to 6 seconds then inhale slowly for 3 to 6 seconds. Repeat this 5 times. Do this whenever you feel a little stressed. It only takes a minute.

Why is breathing good for you? People typically breathe 12 to 20 times a minute at rest. When stressed, people experience fast heart rate and shallow breathing. The diaphragm's range of motion is limited with shallow breathing, resulting in less than fully oxygenated air. Slow, deep breathing encourages full oxygen exchange, improving the chemical balance of the body.

Deep breathing also activates the nervous system and improves the balance between sympathetic and parasympathetic nervous systems, driving heart rate down and lowering blood pressure. Deep breathing has been utilized as a major component of relaxation techniques for stress management, such as yoga and meditation for years. To learn how scientists found the results, see 64, 65, 66, 67 in the reference section. To find more about the breathing benefit, these articles are good and easy to read:

- *Relaxation Techniques for Health* by National Center for Complementary and Integrative Health, NIH: 2014.

- *Relaxation techniques: Breath control helps quell errant stress response* by Harvard Medical School: 2015

- **Deep breathing helps you feel better.**

- **Make it a routine to keep you healthy.**

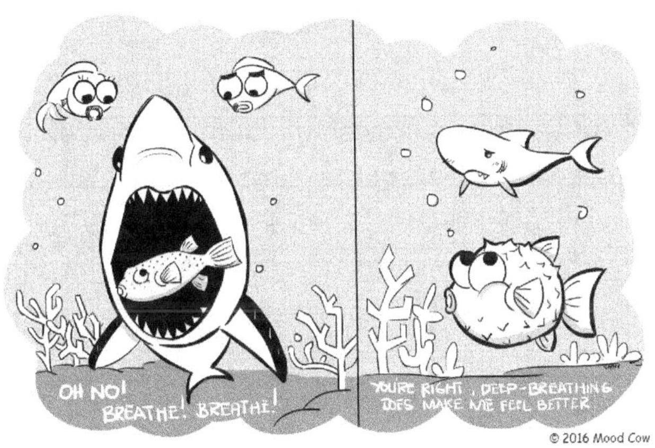

© 2016 Mood Cow

#5 Sleep - Adequate sleep improves health, productivity, and safety.

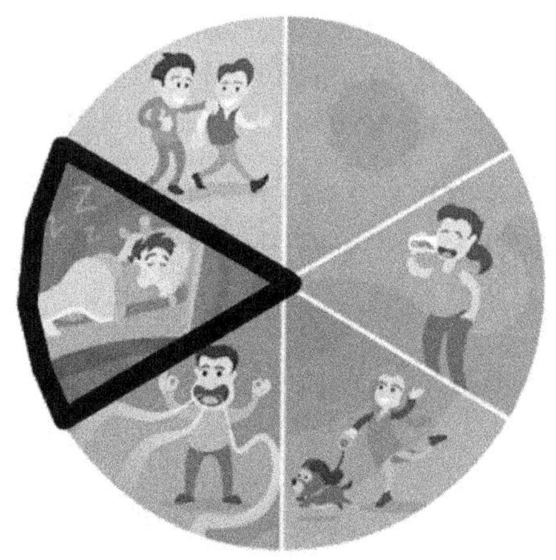

Good restorative sleep is critical for your body and brain. Use the recommended sleep hours in the chart as a guideline to establish your daily regularity. For age 13 to 18 years, 8 to 10 hours of sleep is recommended. A balanced diet, hydration, sunlight and exercise can help you fall asleep and stay asleep longer.

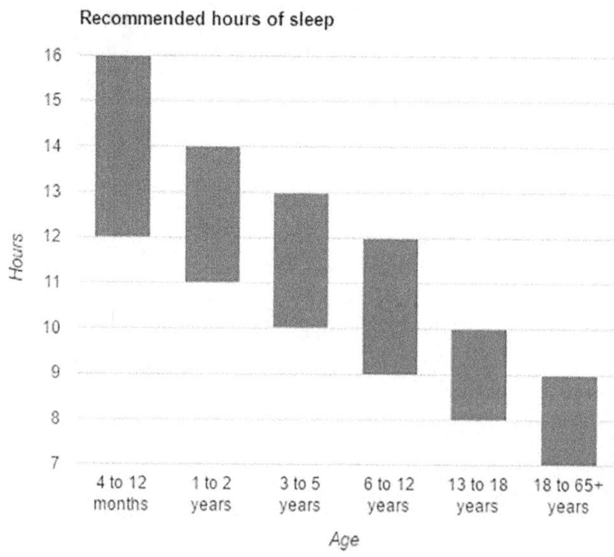

Why is sleep good for you? Insufficient sleep among children and teenagers is a serious health risk. To learn how scientists found the results, see 68, 69, 70, 71, 72 in the reference section. To find more about the sleep benefit, these articles are good and easy to read:

- *Sleep aids: Understand over-the-counter options* by Mayo Clinic: 2014.

- *Sleeping Pills & Natural Sleep Aids: What's Best for You?* by Melinda Smith, Lawrence Robinson, and Robert Segal: 2016.

Caution: If you have problems falling asleep or staying asleep through the night, consult your doctor for advice to improve your sleep. Ask your doctor before taking any medications or supplements.

- **A good night's sleep helps you feel better.**

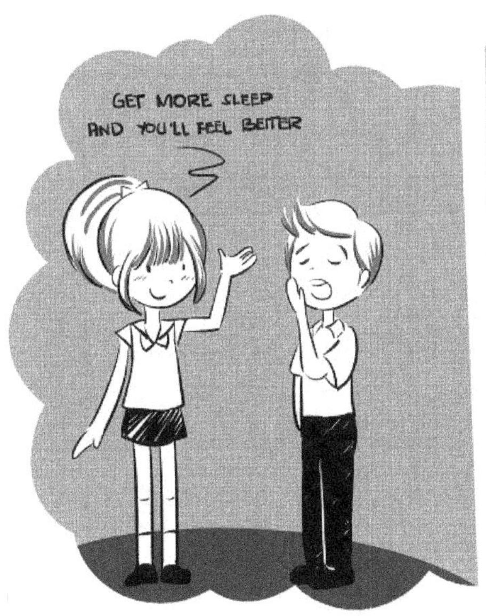

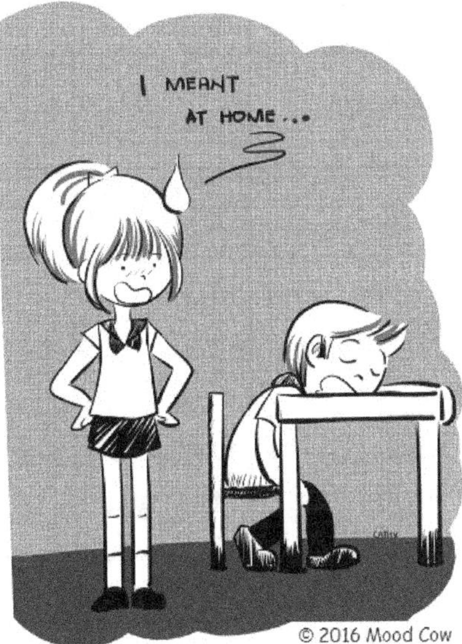

#6 Goodwill - Social and creative activities promote better mental health.

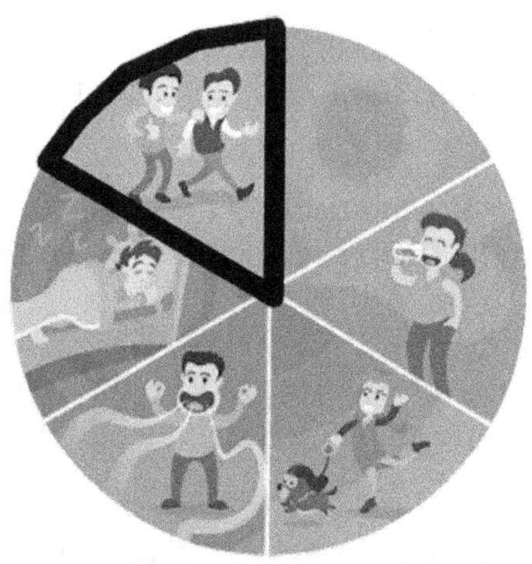

Emotional connection with people and activities can improve your well-being. Give kind, warm, encouraging words and do something nice to your friends, family, colleagues, and even complete strangers.

A good support system is not just your friends and family. It includes your own creative activities. Engage in activities like art, music, dance, drama, writing, poetry, craft works, gardening, cooking, and traveling.

Why is social connection good for you? Evidence in scientific literature indicates that goodwill acts, positive social relationships, and creative activities improve mental wellness. To learn how scientists found the results, see 73, 74, 75, 76, 77 in the reference section. To find more about the connection benefit, these articles are good and easy to read:

- *Teens with upbeat friends may have better emotional health* by Nandini Mani: 2015.

- *Creative Arts Therapy and Expressive Arts Therapy* by Cathy Malchiodi: 2014.

- *How Facebook Makes Us Unhappy* by Maria Konnikova: 2013.

Caution: Be careful with your exposure and involvement in online social relationships. Studies show that social media can have inadvertent but seriously negative effects on mental health.

- **Social connection helps you feel better.**

- **Make it a routine to keep you healthy.**

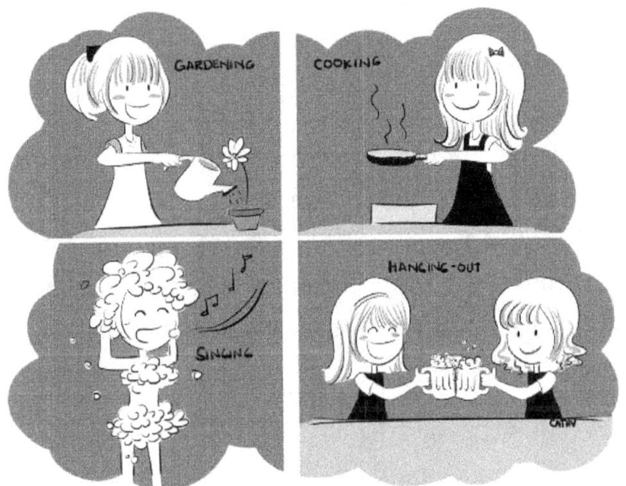

© 2016 Mood Cow

Summary

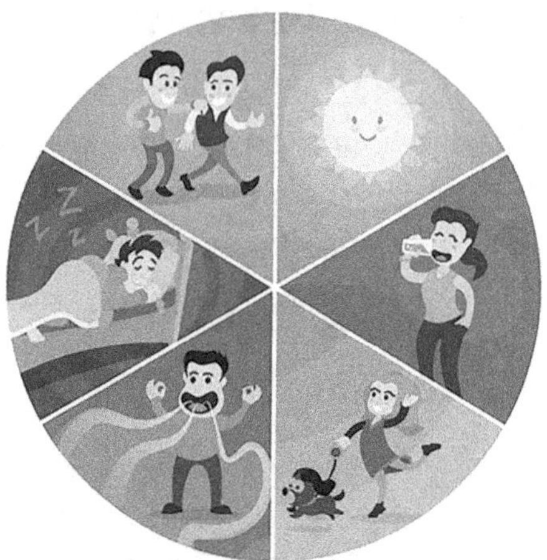

Now you know, simple routines can promote not only physical health but also your mental and emotional health. Even when you think you are doing fine, just remember to take these six actions every day. It's just like brushing teeth or putting hand lotions every night. Your simple daily routine can and will help you avoid problems in the future. Cheers to your good health!

Suggested readings

- *Unraveling the Sun's Role in Depression* by WebMD: 2002. A quick, easy read about sunlight and serotonin benefits. http://www.webmd.com/mental-health/news/20021205/unraveling-suns-role-in-depression

- *Benefits of Sunlight: A Bright Spot for Human Health* by M. Nathaniel Mead: 2008. A broad, scientific narration on sunlight benefits. https://www.ncbi.nlm.nih.gov/pmc/articles/PMC2290997/

- *Even Mild Dehydration Can Alter Mood* by Colin Poitras: 2012. An easy read about the research behind hydration. http://today.uconn.edu/2012/02/even-mild-dehydration-can-alter-mood/

- *From bad breath to car accidents, dehydration is a real health threat* by Linda Melone: 2015. A CNN article on the importance of hydration. http://www.cnn.com/2015/06/01/health/dehydration-body/

- *Food to Balance Your Mood* by Star Lawrence: 2002. A WebMD article on the importance of eating the right food. http://www.webmd.com/food-recipes/features/food-to-balance-your-mood#1

- *The Mental Health Benefits of Exercise* by L. Robinson, J. Segal, and M. Smith: 2016. An easy guidebook on how to get started on your own exercise plan. http://www.helpguide.org/articles/exercise-fitness/emotional-benefits-of-exercise.htm Link

- *Relaxation Techniques for Health* by National Center for Complementary and Integrative Health, NIH: 2014. This article is well-grounded in current science and offers a broad view of relaxation techniques. https://nccih.nih.gov/health/stress/relaxation.htm

- *Relaxation techniques: Breath control helps quell errant stress response* by Harvard Medical School: 2015. A practical guide to deep breathing. http://www.health.harvard.edu/mind-and-mood/relaxation-techniques-breath-control-helps-quell-errant-stress-response

- *Sleep aids: Understand over-the-counter options* by Mayo Clinic: 2014. Read this quick guide from Mayo Clinic before you try any medication. http://www.mayoclinic.org/healthy-lifestyle/adult-health/in-depth/sleep-aids/art-20047860

- *Sleeping Pills & Natural Sleep Aids: What's Best for You?* by Melinda Smith, Lawrence Robinson, and Robert Segal: 2016. Another good read on sleeping pills. http://www.helpguide.org/articles/sleep/sleeping-pills-and-natural-sleep-aids.htm

- *Sleep and mental health* by Harvard Medical School: 2009 A well-written article on sleep problems and mental health. http://www.health.harvard.edu/newsletter_article/Sleep-and-mental-health

- *Teens with upbeat friends may have better emotional health* by Nandini Mani: 2015. A good article on new studies regarding the benefits of having positive friends. http://www.health.harvard.edu/blog/teens-with-upbeat-friends-may-have-better-emotional-health-201512108797

- *Creative Arts Therapy and Expressive Arts Therapy* by Cathy Malchiodi: 2014. A good overview of creative interventions used in psychotherapies. https://www.psychologytoday.com/blog/arts-and-health/201406/creative-arts-therapy-and-expressive-arts-therapy

- *How Facebook Makes Us Unhappy* by Maria Konnikova: 2013. A New Yorker article on the negative effects of online social media. http://www.newyorker.com/tech/elements/how-facebook-makes-us-unhappy

References

57. Kent ST, McClure LA, Crosson WL, Arnett DK, Wadley VG, Sathiakumar N. Effect of sunlight exposure on cognitive function among depressed and non-depressed participants: a REGARDS cross-sectional study. Environmental Health. 2009;8:34. https://www.ncbi.nlm.nih.gov/pmc/articles/PMC2728098/

58. Lam RW, Levitt AJ, Levitan RD, et al. Efficacy of Bright Light Treatment, Fluoxetine, and the Combination in Patients With Nonseasonal Major Depressive Disorder: A Randomized Clinical Trial. JAMA Psychiatry. 2016;73(1):56-63. http://jamanetwork.com/journals/jamapsychiatry/article-abstract/2470681

59. Lieverse R, Van Someren EW, Nielen MA, Uitdehaag BJ, Smit JH, Hoogendijk WG. Bright Light Treatment in Elderly Patients With Nonseasonal Major Depressive Disorder: A Randomized Placebo-Controlled Trial. Arch Gen Psychiatry. 2011;68(1):61-70. http://jamanetwork.com/journals/jamapsychiatry/fullarticle/211002

60. Brandis K., Fluid Physiology, Ch3.1 Water Turnover. http://www.anaesthesiamcq.com/FluidBook/fl3_1.php

61. Ganio MS, Armstrong LE, Casa DJ, McDermott BP, Lee EC, Yamamoto LM, Marzano S, Lopez RM, Jimenez L, Bellego LL, Chevillotte E, Lieberman HR. Mild dehydration impairs cognitive performance and mood of men. British Journal of Nutrition. 2011;106(1) :1535-1543. https://www.cambridge.org/core/journals/british-journal-of-nutrition/article/mild-dehydration-impairs-cognitive-performance-and-mood-of-men/3388AB36B8DF73E844C9AD19271A75BF

62. Rao TSS, Asha MR, Ramesh BN, Rao KSJ. Understanding nutrition, depression and mental illnesses. Indian Journal of Psychiatry. 2008;50(2):77-82. https://www.ncbi.nlm.nih.gov/pmc/articles/PMC2738337/

63. Physical Activity Guidelines Advisory Committee Report, Part G. Section 8: Mental Health, Office of Disease Prevention and Health Promotion, 2016. https://health.gov/paguidelines/report/G8_mentalhealth.aspx

64. Cabral P, Meyer HB, Ames D. Effectiveness of Yoga Therapy as a Complementary Treatment for Major Psychiatric Disorders: A Meta-Analysis. The Primary Care Companion to CNS Disorders. 2011;13(4). https://www.ncbi.nlm.nih.gov/pmc/articles/PMC3219516/

65. Chiesa A., Serretti A. Mindfulness-Based Stress Reduction for Stress Management in Healthy People: A Review and Meta-Analysis. The Journal of Alternative and Complementary Medicine. May 2009;15(5): 593-600. http://online.liebertpub.com/doi/abs/10.1089/acm.2008.0495

66. Grossman P., Niemann L., Schmidt S., Walach H. Mindfulness-based stress reduction and health benefits: A meta-analysis. Journal of Psychosomatic Research 2004;57: 35–43. http://online.liebertpub.com/doi/abs/10.1089/acm.2008.0495

67. Spijkerman, MPJ., Pots, WTM., Bohlmeijer, ET. Effectiveness of online mindfulness-based interventions in improving mental health: A review and meta-analysis of randomised controlled trials. Clinical Psychology Review. 2016. http://www.sciencedirect.com/science/article/pii/S0272735815300623

68. Paruthi S, Brooks LJ, D'Ambrosio C, Hall WA, Kotagal S, Lloyd RM, Malow BA, Maski K, Nichols C, Quan SF, Rosen CL, Troester MM, Wise MS. Recommended amount of sleep for pediatric populations: a consensus statement of the American Academy of Sleep Medicine. J Clin Sleep Med 2016;12(6):785–786. http://www.aasmnet.org/articles.aspx?id=6326

69. Hirshkowitz, M. et al. National Sleep Foundation's sleep time duration recommendations: methodology and results summary. Sleep Health: Journal of the National Sleep Foundation. 2015;1:40-43. http://www.sleephealthjournal.org/article/S2352-7218(15)00015-7/fulltext

70. Institute of Medicine, Committee on Sleep Medicine and Research. Sleep disorders and sleep deprivation: An unmet public health problem. Washington: National Academies Press; 2006. https://www.ncbi.nlm.nih.gov/books/NBK19960/

71. Centers for Disease Control and Prevention, Epidemiology Program Office. Perceived insufficient rest or sleep among adults: United States, 2008. MMWR. 2009 Oct 30;58(42):1175-9. http://www.cdc.gov/mmwr/preview/mmwrhtml/mm5842a2.htm

72. Schutte-Rodin S, Broch L, Buysse D, Dorsey C, Sateia M. Clinical Guideline for the Evaluation and Management of Chronic Insomnia in Adults. Journal of Clinical Sleep Medicine: Official Publication of the American Academy of Sleep Medicine. 2008;4(5):487-504. https://www.ncbi.nlm.nih.gov/pmc/articles/PMC2576317/

73. Umberson D, Montez JK. Social Relationships and Health: A Flashpoint for Health Policy. Journal of health and social behavior. 2010;51(Suppl):S54-S66. https://www.ncbi.nlm.nih.gov/pmc/articles/PMC3150158/

74. Hill EM., Griffiths FE, House T. Spreading of healthy mood in adolescent social networks. Proc. R. Soc. B 2015 August 19; 282: 20151180. http://rspb.royalsocietypublishing.org/content/282/1813/20151180/

75. Siedliecki SL, Good M. Effect of music on power, pain, depression and disability. Journal of Advanced Nursing. 2006;54: 553–562. https://www.ncbi.nlm.nih.gov/pubmed/16722953

76. Gussak D. The effectiveness of art therapy in reducing depression in prison populations. Int J Offender Ther Comp Criminol. 2007 Aug;51(4):444-60. https://www.ncbi.nlm.nih.gov/pubmed/17652148

77. Meekums B, Karkou V, Nelson EA. Dance movement therapy for depression. Cochrane Database Syst Rev. 2015 Feb 19;2:CD009895. https://www.ncbi.nlm.nih.gov/pubmed/25695871

BEST FIRST RESOURCES FOR SELF-HELP

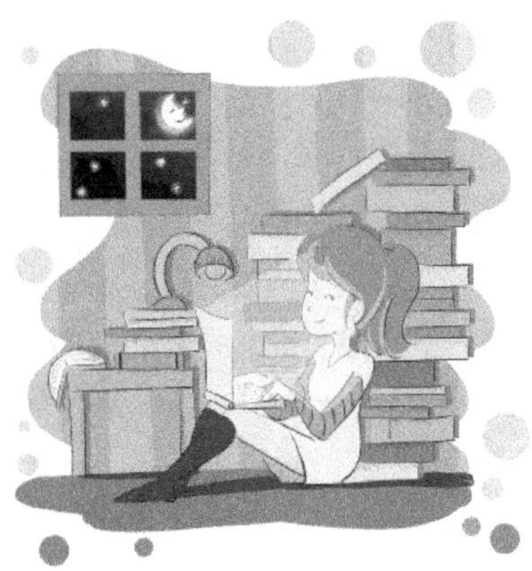

IF YOU LOOK around and search for self-help, you'll quickly discover that there are massive numbers and varieties of self-help resources out there. All self-help products are informational in nature and employ a particular strategy or combination of them to help stimulate, relax, or regulate your problems.

For example, diet self-help uses biochemical and physical modes; yoga and meditation self-help use sensory, physical, and spiritual modes; and motivational self-help uses the cognitive mode.

Leaning toward a particular mode is a personal choice, but a balanced mixture of all six would be ideal.

Self-help products can be classified into four categories.

Reference: This is a purely informational resource, mostly available in books and on websites. Commonly covered topics are medications, diagnostics, treatment, and services available for further action.

Self-assessment: Some books, websites, and mobile apps present information on how to assess certain conditions such as depression and anxiety. They present self-diagnostic tests or questions for readers to assess themselves.

Self-treatment: This problem-solving resource goes a step beyond assessment to make claims for treatment. Diet guidebooks are a good example of this type. They tend to make claims about how a particular activity or substance helps people solve problems or accomplish goals, along with anecdotal stories to support their claims. They then extend their applicability to the general public with some disclaimers in fine print.

Communities: This resource connects people who share similar experiences. Self-help groups can include face-to-face meet-ups, or an online forum.

The best first resource

In this chapter, the best first resources are chosen for each category: reference, self-assessment, self-treatment, and communities. You can use this as a benchmark to compare with your search results. The idea is to start with a big picture first using a broad perspective, then zoom in to more focused resources to meet your specific needs and preferences. This process itself is a cognitive mode of self-help, which is good for you.

B.1. The best first reference

The best first reference book

American Medical Association Family Medical Guide

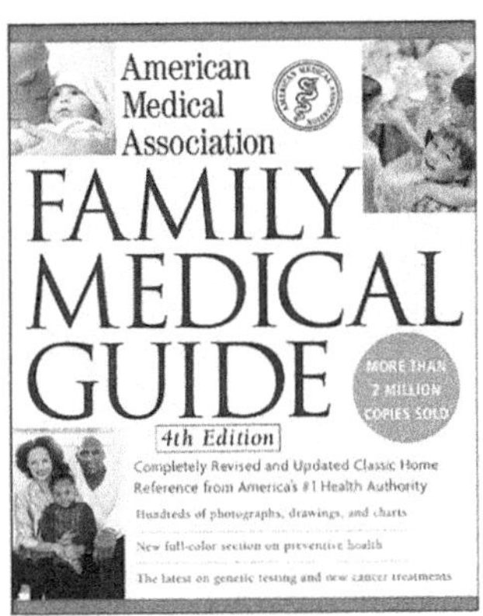

It's safe to say that recent advances in neuroscience finally allow us to think of mental health as a biochemical condition of the brain, not an illness of the mind. From this scientific perspective, it is best to have a general reference book on the health of our entire body. You'll learn that physical, mental, and social conditions are all related in influencing your overall well-being.

People these days may find printed books archaic, but think again. A printed resource is still valuable because you can browse through the content at your leisure and often discover things that you may not otherwise find, especially in large volume books. Seeing visual images in print and feeling the texture of paper offer a sensory mode of self-help as stimulating and relaxing.

This particular book was chosen as the best first reference book because:

- The content is comprehensive and well-balanced between physical and mental health.

- It is ranked and rated highly by users at various online bookstores.

- It is written and published by one of the most credible organizations, the American Medical Association.

- The price is lower than other similar reference books.

The best first reference website

PsychCentral.com

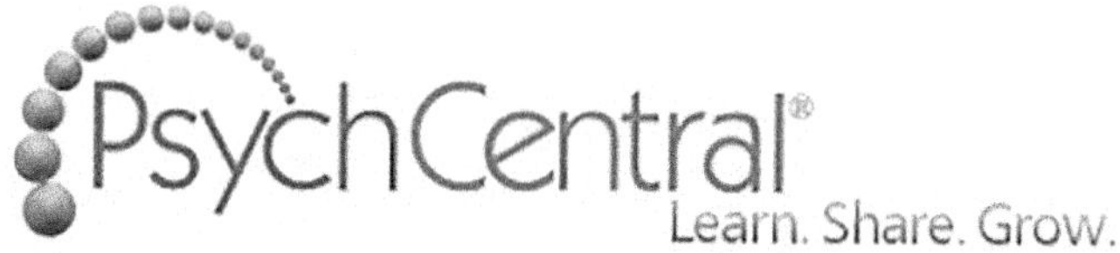

https://psychcentral.com/

While printed forms of reference are good, most people prefer online resources so that they can access information as needed on more topic-focused materials. There is one website that stands out from all the others — PsychCentral.com. It started before the explosion of the World Wide Web and continues its tradition of gathering and updating relevant content as reference materials on mental health.

This particular website was chosen as the best first resource website because:

- The content is more comprehensive than any other site.

- The content is neutral and not biased toward any particular product, treatment, theory, or policy.

- The content is constantly updated and supervised by its founder and editor, Dr. John Grohol.

- It is ranked and rated highly by users and media.

- All the content is free.

The best first reference mobile app

None.

Unfortunately, there is no recommended mobile app as the go-to reference resource for mental health at this time. An increasing number of apps are available in the market, but many of them are focused on specific symptoms or problems.

PsychCentral has an iPhone app, but not one for Android. The good news is that you can use your mobile browser to access PsychCentral.com. The downside is that you need a network connection to access it.

B.2. The best first self-assessment resource

The best first self-assessment book

DSM, the Diagnostic and Statistical Manual of Mental Disorders

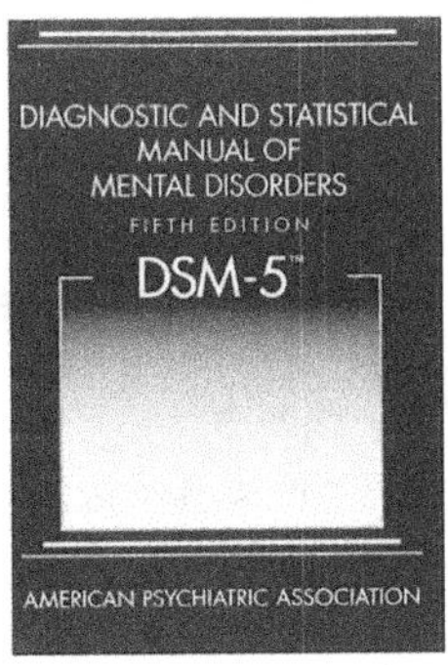

Self-assessment these days implies personality and skill testing for corporate human resource and personnel management. If this is where your interest lies, there is no book to recommend. But if you are wondering whether your particular psychiatric conditions fit the definition or criteria of mental illness, I have an extraordinary resource to recommend.

The Diagnostic and Statistical Manual of Mental Disorders (DSM) is not an ordinary book. Published by the American Psychiatric Association, this is the universal authority in the US for psychiatric diagnosis, treatment recommendations, and insurance payment criteria. Clinicians, drug manufacturers, insurance companies, policymakers, lawyers, and researchers all rely on DSM.

DSM is important, not because of its scientific accuracy, but because of its authoritative power. If your conditions don't fit any of the defined diseases, your treatment may not be covered by your health insurance. If you are going to do self-assessment, you might as well use the same source that your doctor uses.

A word of caution is in order when using DSM. DSM is definitive only in the sense of its standardized use in this country. The psychiatric diagnostic categories are still subjective and symptom-based. In other words, readers are advised to use DSM for the purpose of understanding how psychiatric illnesses are defined, and how the way you present your symptoms to doctors affect their decisions on diagnosis, treatment, and insurance coverage. DSM is excellent for this purpose.

This particular book was chosen as the best first self-assessment book because:

- It is the single authoritative resource in psychiatry, published by the American Psychiatric Association.

- The content provides comprehensive diagnostic criteria for current psychiatric illnesses.

- It is accessible, though expensive and hard to use, by the general public.

The best first self-assessment website

MedlinePlus, Mental Health and Behavior Section

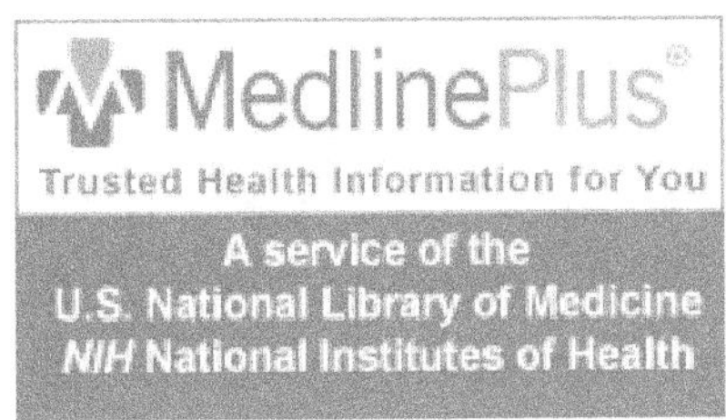

https://medlineplus.gov/mentalhealthandbehavior.html

Most people are on the lookout for more accessible and readable materials than DSM-5. MedlinePlus is designed specifically for that purpose. This website is run by the US National Library of Medicine to provide information about diseases and conditions in language that the general public can understand.

The mental health and behavior section of MedlinePlus covers broad topics in mental health in a well-organized way. It even covers topics that are not commonly addressed by other general websites, such as dementia, phobia, and self-harm, with reliable links to further resources.

This particular website was chosen as the best first self-assessment website because:

- The content is more comprehensive than other sites.

- The content is written and updated by the US Library of Medicine.

- The content has many links to reliable resources for further exploration.

- All the content is free.

The best first self-assessment mobile app

None.

Despite the large number of apps in the market, it is disappointing that no mobile app qualifies as the best first resource for self-assessment other than the app version of DSM-5. Most apps use micro-assessment tools, such as depression tests, anxiety tests, and stress tests in the form of questionnaires. As self-help, such isolated assessment processes are inadequate unless they accompany thorough explanation and further exploratory information.

Clinicians are struggling with the lack of efficacy of mobile apps. This article may shed some light on the subject.

https://psychcentral.com/news/2016/04/27/guidelines-help-clinicians-evaluate-mobile-apps/102397.html

Just like the printed version of DSM-5, the mobile app version of DSM-5 is expensive ($69). You can use MedlinePlus in your mobile browser when you have a network connection.

B.3. The best first self-treatment resource

The best first self-treatment book

Little Book of Mindfulness by Patricia Collard, 2014

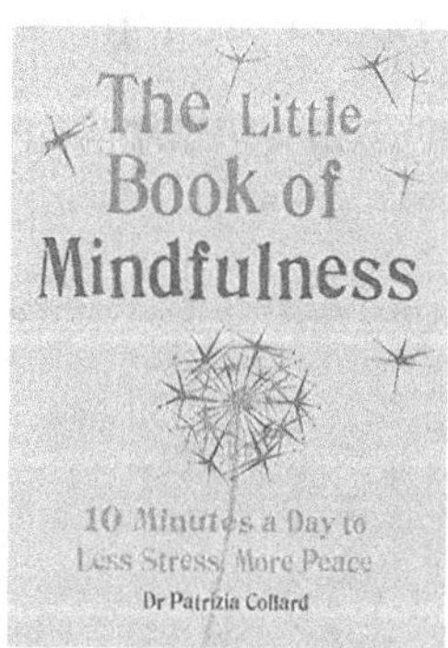

Unlike reference and self-assessment materials that need to be comprehensive and precise, the primary self-treatment resource needs to be approachable and practical for the general public to accommodate a variety of circumstances. Many self-help books are long and tedious, requiring tremendous mental focus and effort to digest.

This short book (only 96 pages) shows simple 5- to 10-minute practices to relieve stress and raise awareness of oneself. The concept is based on the currently popular ideas of cognitive behavioral therapy (CBT) and mindfulness. The easy, practical, and visual nature of the book makes it not only approachable, but also adds sensory and physical modes of self-help.

There should be an underlying assumption that the efficacy of self-help treatment is limited unless there is the collaborative support of healthcare professionals. Because the book is based on CBT and mindfulness, which are already clinically shown to be effective, what you learn from this book is applicable and extendable to other self-help methods.

This particular book was chosen as the best first self-treatment book because:

- The content is based on cognitive, behavioral, and mindfulness concepts.

- The content is generalized for further application and exploration.

- The content is short and written in easy-to-read language.

- The book is rated highly by users.

- The book is inexpensive (US$8 print, US$2 digital) and easily accessible.

The best first self-treatment website

HelpGuide.org

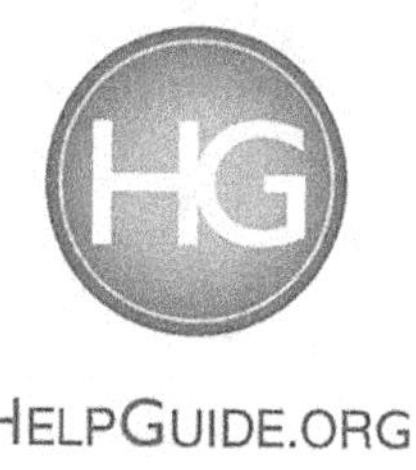

HELPGUIDE.ORG

https://www.helpguide.org/

What differentiates websites from books and mobile apps is flexibility and real estate that allow for the creative packaging and delivery of complex information. HelpGuide.org is an excellent example of a creative compilation of information as actionable knowledge. Self-help is about action, and this website understands and executes this very well. Because of that, HelpGuide is the best first self-treatment website.

The site covers a wide range of topics with a consistent and visually pleasing structure. Every topic contains actionable information that gives the reader hope and motivation to act. Often neglected but increasingly important topics such as caregiving, grandparenting, aging well, and senior housing are addressed.

This particular website was chosen as the best first self-treatment site because:

- The content has broad coverage with actionable information as self-help.

- The content is generalized for further application and exploration.

- The content is well-structured and visually pleasing.

The best first self-treatment mobile app

Headspace

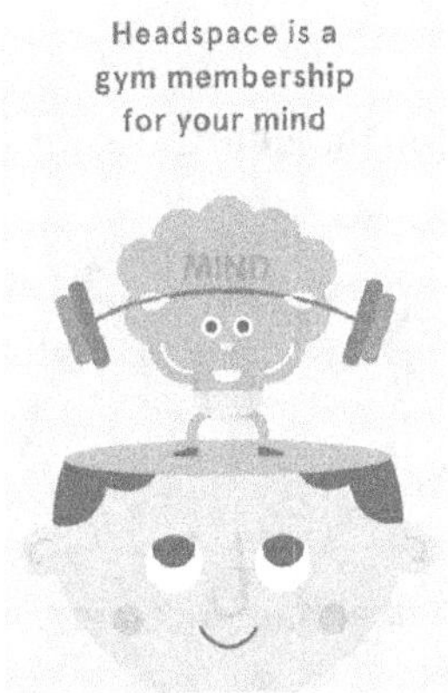

https://www.headspace.com/

There are thousands of mobile apps for mental health self-treatment, but there is no evidence supporting how effective they are. Still, their usability has been evaluated based on MARS (mobile application rating scale). A group of researchers in Australia looked at 700 mindfulness apps and rated 23 for their usability. Headspace received the highest with a score of 4.0 out of 5.0.[1]

This particular app was chosen as the best first self-treatment app because:

- The content is based on mindfulness concepts.

- The app is one of the most downloaded apps (over one million downloads).

- The app is rated highly by users.

- The usability has been evaluated and rated highest by independent research.

---

1   Mani M. Kavanagh DJ. Hides L. Stoyanov SR. Review and Evaluation of Mindfulness-Based iPhone Apps. *JMIR Mhealth Uhealth*. 2015 Aug 19;3(3):e82. https://www.ncbi.nlm.nih.gov/pubmed/26290327

B.4. The best first community resource

The best first support community: Support Groups Listing

Mental Health America

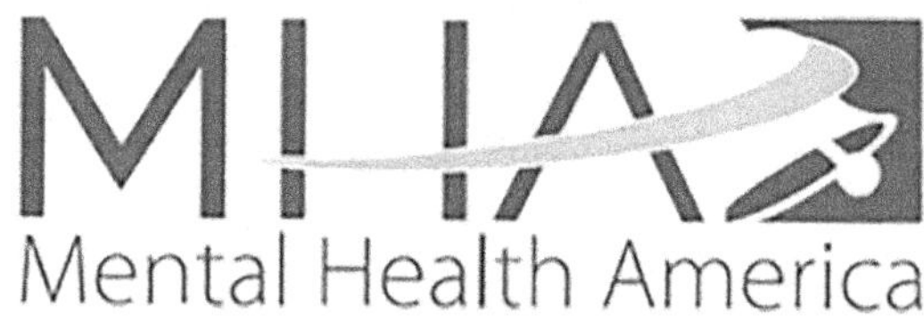

http://www.mentalhealthamerica.net/find-support-groups

Your experience is valuable knowledge that can help other people. Meeting as a group or in an online forum is a good social and cognitive mode of self-help. You can learn from them, and they can learn from you.

Mental Health America (MHA) has a long list of various support groups on its website. You can browse through them to locate one to fit your needs and find out if the organization has an online forum or local support group near you.

The best first support community: Online Community

PsychCentral Support Community

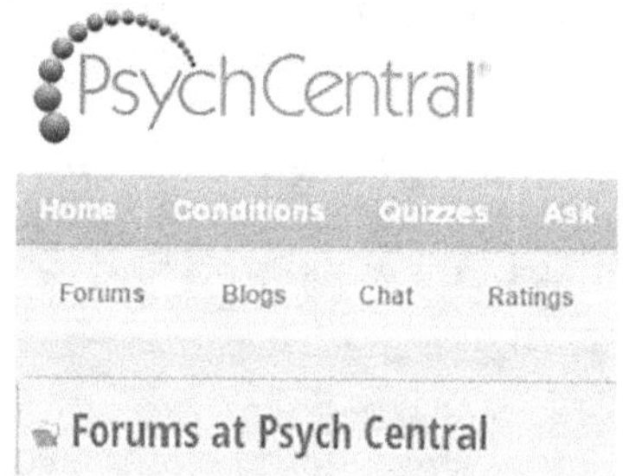

https://forums.psychcentral.com/

An online forum is the quickest, easiest way to take advantage of the social mode of self-help. You gain access to hundreds of thousands of posts from people asking and answering questions, making comments, and sharing their knowledge and experience.

PsychCentral hosts the oldest and largest online community on mental health. This is the best first resource because:

- The forum is the oldest, largest, and most used community since 1991.

- The community has almost 400,000 members and over 5 million posts.

- The community covers a wide variety of topics and subtopics.

- The site is maintained by one of the most trusted sources, PsychCentral.

The best first support community: Mobile apps

7 Cups of Tea

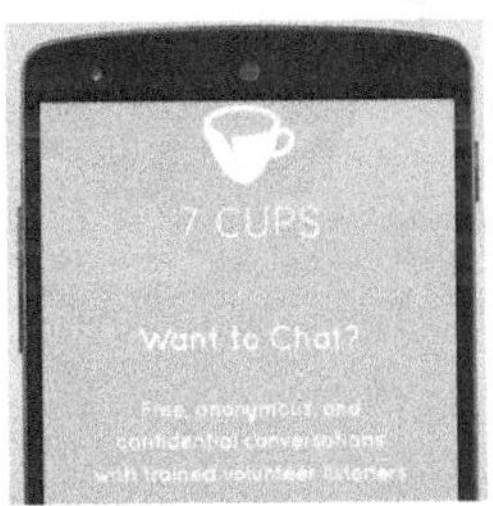

https://www.7cups.com/

7 Cups of Tea offers a new kind of social support that differs from typical online forums or tele-therapists. This new service works very well on a mobile device platform, and that's why it's the best first mobile community app.

7 Cups of Tea hosts a group of volunteers called "listeners." You will be automatically connected to one of these listeners at random,

and you can chat about whatever you feel like. The listeners are not therapists. They are simply people out there willing to listen to you and chat a little bit.

The concept seems to work well on mobile devices as people are used to text messaging. Often it seems intimidating to talk to a therapist, and you have to guard yourself on online forums, as they leave traces of what you write. A casual chat with a complete stranger may be exactly what you need to fulfill your social wants. 7 Cups of Tea has a standard forum for threaded conversations as well as some calming activities.

This particular app was chosen as the best first community app because:

- It offers a non-intimidating, casual chat function that no other app provides.

- The app also hosts online communities.

- The app has a relatively large number of downloads with high ratings from users.

SUGGESTED LESSON MATERIALS AT HOME

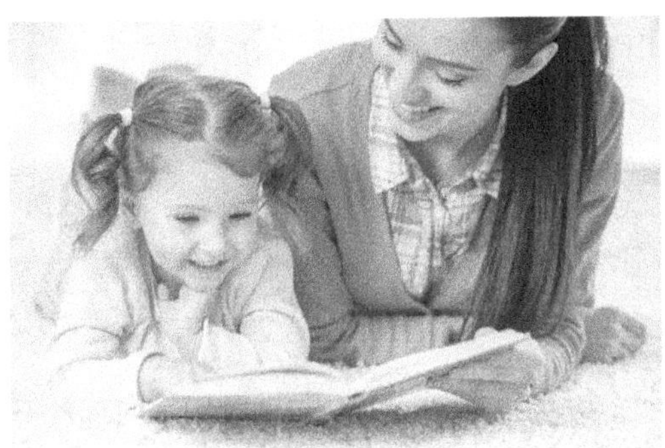

BOOKS ARE GREAT tools for parents and children to share stories, ideas, lessons, and most importantly, quality time together. In this chapter, some useful books and materials are compiled for the early childhood mental care curriculum as outlined in Chapter 6.

Topic 1: How you feel — the skill to recognize and verbalize emotion

The first topic of the curriculum is about feelings. We want our children to recognize different types of feelings and verbalize their feelings in words. The ability to recognize and verbalize feelings is an important social skill for young children. It gives them a healthier way to express themselves than resorting to poor behavior that often arises from emotional stress. It promotes constructive social environment through communication with others. In addition, as evidenced in neuroscience, putting feelings into words reduces the effect of stressors, and helps children manage their negative emotional experiences.

Lessons about feelings and emotions are fairly commonly addressed by many authors and educators for young children. However, there aren't many materials that specifically identify and teach children how feelings and behaviors are related, and how to recognize other people's feelings. Fortunately, I found some helpful books for your home use.

Lesson 1: Different types of feelings

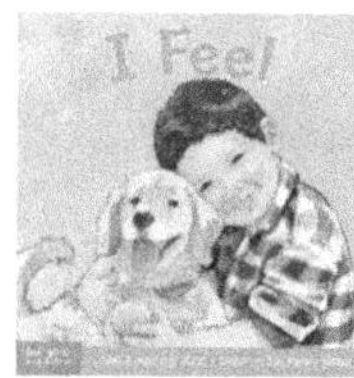

"I Feel" by Cheri J. Meiners, M.Ed. / illustrated by Penny Weber, Free Spirit Publishing Inc., Minneapolis, MN. ISBN: 978-1-63198-217-0, Page count: 24, Price: less than $10. https://www.freespirit.com/early-childhood/i-feel-learning-about-me-and-you-cheri-meiners-penny-weber

Lesson 2: Feelings and behaviors

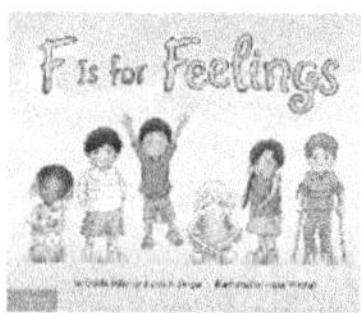

"F Is for Feelings" by Goldie Millar, Ph.D. and Lisa Berger, Ph.D. / illustrated by Hazel Mitchell, Free Spirit Publishing Inc., Minneapolis, MN. ISBN: 978-1-57542-476-7 (paperback) / ISBN: 978-1-57542-475-0 (hardcover), Page count: 40, Price: less than $20. https://www.freespirit.com/early-childhood/f-is-for-feelings-goldie-millar-lisa-berger/

Lesson 3: Good ways and bad ways to express feelings

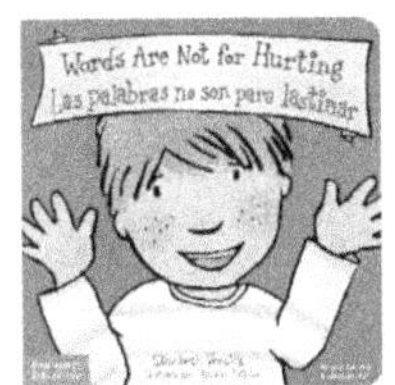

"Words Are Not for Hurting" by Elizabeth Verdick / illustrated by Marieka Heinlen, Free Spirit Publishing Inc., Minneapolis, MN. ISBN: 978-1-57542-311-1, Page count: 24, Price: less than $10. https://www.freespirit.com/early-childhood/words-are-not-for-hurting-las-palabras-no-son-para-lastimar-board-book-best-behavior-elizabeth-verdick-marieka-heinlen/

Lesson 4: Feelings of other people

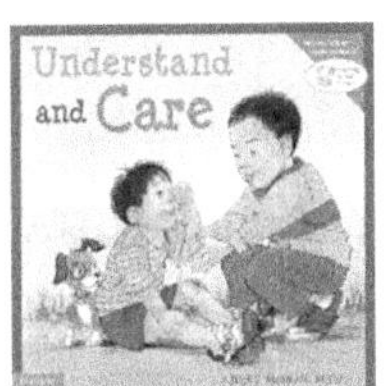

"Understand and Care" by Cheri J. Meiners, M.Ed. / illustrated by Meredith Johnson, Free Spirit Publishing Inc., Minneapolis, MN. ISBN: 978-1-57542-131-5, Page count: 40, Price: about $10. https://www.freespirit.com/early-childhood/understand-and-care-learning-to-get-along-cheri-meiners/

Lesson 5: Teasing and bullying

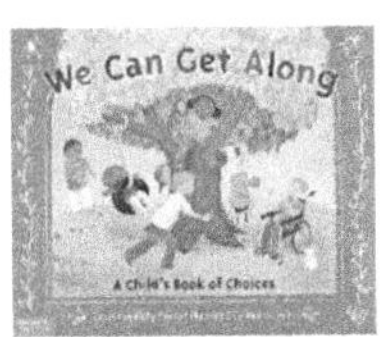

"We Can Get Along" by Lauren Murphy Payne, M.S.W. / illustrated by Melissa Iwai, Free Spirit Publishing Inc., Minneapolis, MN. ISBN: 978-1-63198-027-5 (paperback) / ISBN: 978-1-63198-049-7 (hardcover), Page count: 40, Price: about $10. https://www.freespirit.com/early-childhood/we-can-get-along-lauren-murphy-payne-melissa-iwai/

For older children 5+

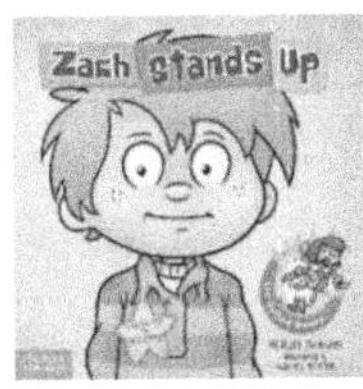

"Zach Stands Up" by William Mulcahy / illustrated by Darren McKee, Free Spirit Publishing Inc., Minneapolis, MN. ISBN: 978-1-63198-293-4,

Page count: 36, Price: about $10. https://www.freespirit.com/early-childhood/zach-stands-up-william-mulcahy-darren-mckee

Topic 2: What makes you feel certain ways — the skill to recognize influencers

As the first topic addressed the "what" part of feelings, the second topic moves on to the "why" part of feelings. We want **both children and parents** to recognize certain things that are uplifting and make you feel positive, and certain things that are downers and make you feel negative. The ability to recognize the positive and negative influencers is an important social skill, potentially more important than the feeling itself. Knowing what helps them feel, think, and behave better in the presence of stress builds resilience in children. It also promotes healthy relationships between children and parents. This is advocated by both developmental science of early childhood and the World Health Organization.

Unfortunately, there aren't many books and materials that directly teach this topic. We want to talk about various influencers in physical, social, and mental elements. Perhaps parents can use the materials in the Topic 1 again, and reframe the discussion with children to focus on the following five lesson themes:

- **Lesson 6:** Influencers in family and school
- **Lesson 7:** Influencers in TV, movies, music, video games
- **Lesson 8:** Influence by weather, food, and outdoor activities
- **Lesson 9:** Influence by illness and injury
- **Lesson 10:** Other influencers

The following three books may be useful.

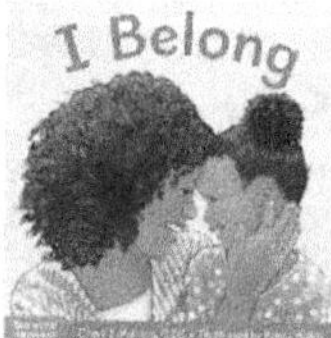

"I Belong" by Cheri J. Meiners, M.Ed. / illustrated by Penny Weber, Free Spirit Publishing Inc., Minneapolis, MN. ISBN: 978-1-63198-214-9, Page count: 24, Price: about $10. https://www.freespirit.

com/early-childhood/i-belong-learning-about-me-and-you-cheri-meiners-penny-weber

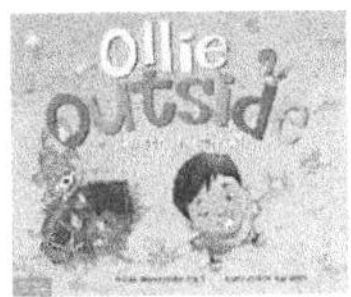

"Ollie Outside: Screen-Free Fun" by Michael Oberschneider, Psy.D. / illustrated by Guy Wolek, Free Spirit Publishing Inc., Minneapolis, MN., ISBN: 978-1-63198-068-8 (paperback) / ISBN: 978-1-63198-105-0 (hardcover), Page count: 32, Price: about $10. https://www.freespirit.com/early-childhood/ollie-outside-michael-oberschneider-guy-wolek

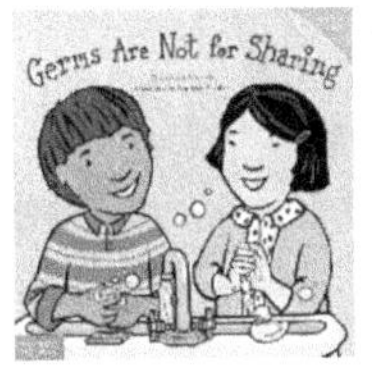

"Germs Are Not for Sharing" by Elizabeth Verdick / illustrated by Marieka Heinlen, Free Spirit Publishing Inc., Minneapolis, MN., ISBN: 978-1-57542-197-1, Page count: 40, Price: about $10. https://www.freespirit.com/early-childhood/germs-are-not-for-sharing-paperback-best-behavior-elizabeth-verdick-marieka-heinlen/

Topic 3: How to self-calm and communicate — the skill to self-calm and communicate for help

With the new skills about what and why of feelings, children can advance to the "how" part of feelings. Understanding how the social rules and manners work, children can gain confidence in expressing their feelings properly and communicating with adults for help. But before they can communicate, they first need to know how to calm themselves down. Here are some useful books to teach children how to self-calm, communicate, and make good choices.

Lesson 11: Self-help and self-calming

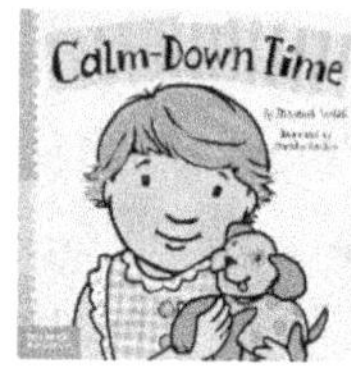 **"Calm-Down Time"** by Elizabeth Verdick / illustrated by Marieka Heinlen, Free Spirit Publishing Inc., Minneapolis, MN., ISBN: 978-1-57542-316-6, Page count: 24, Price: less than $10. https://www.freespirit.com/early-childhood/calm-down-time-toddler-tools-elizabeth-verdick-marieka-heinlen/

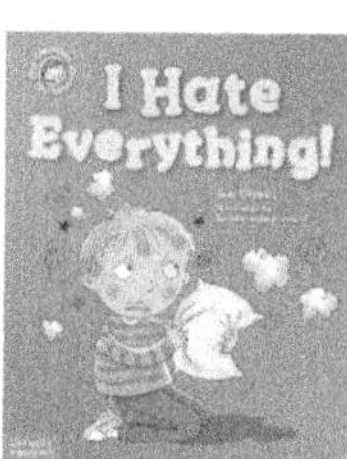 **"I Hate Everything! A book about feeling angry"** by Sue Graves / illustrated by Desideria Guicciardini, Free Spirit Publishing Inc., Minneapolis, MN., ISBN: 978-1-57542-443-9, Page count: 28, Price: about $10. https://www.freespirit.com/early-childhood/i-hate-everything-our-emotions-and-behavior-sue-graves-desideria-guicciardini/

Lesson 12: Attention, look, and listen

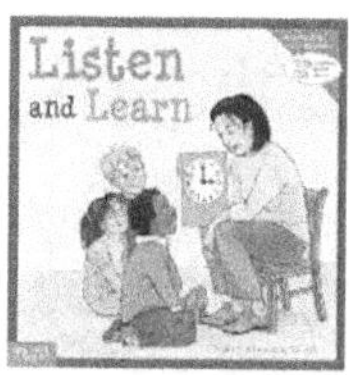 **"Listen and Learn"** by Cheri J. Meiners, M.Ed. / illustrated by Meredith Johnson, Free Spirit Publishing Inc., Minneapolis, MN., ISBN: 978-1-57542-123-0, Page count: 40, Price: about $10. https://www.freespirit.com/early-childhood/listen-and-learn-learning-to-get-along-cheri-meiners/

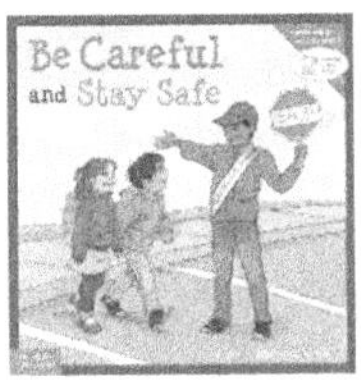

"Be Careful and Stay Safe" by Cheri J. Meiners, M.Ed. / illustrated by Meredith Johnson, Free Spirit Publishing Inc., Minneapolis, MN., ISBN: 978-1-57542-211-4, Page count: 40, Price: about $10. https://www.freespirit.com/early-childhood/be-careful-and-stay-safe-learning-to-get-along-cheri-meiners/

Lesson 13: Help at home, school, and community

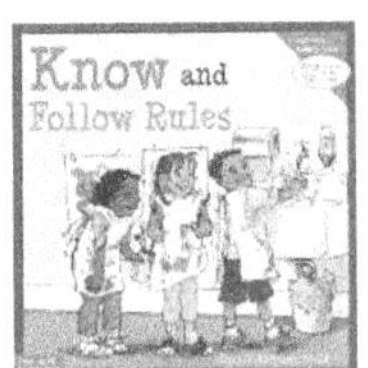

"Know and Follow Rules" by Cheri J. Meiners, M.Ed. / illustrated by Meredith Johnson, Free Spirit Publishing Inc., Minneapolis, MN., ISBN: 978-1-57542-130-8, Page count: 40, Price: about $10. https://www.freespirit.com/early-childhood/know-and-follow-rules-learning-to-get-along-cheri-meiners/

Lesson 14: Needs, wants, feelings

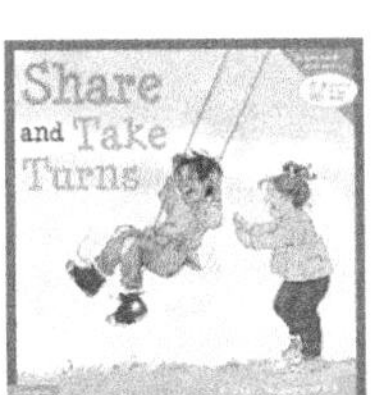

"Share and Take Turns" by Cheri J. Meiners, M.Ed. / illustrated by Meredith Johnson, Free Spirit Publishing Inc., Minneapolis, MN., ISBN: 978-1-57542-124-7, Page count: 40, Price: about $10. https://www.freespirit.com/early-childhood/share-and-take-turns-learning-to-get-along-cheri-meiners/

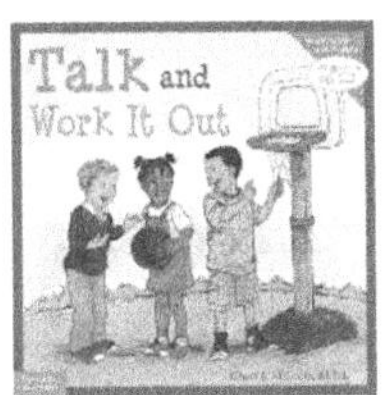

"Talk and Work It Out" by Cheri J. Meiners, M.Ed. / illustrated by Meredith Johnson, Free Spirit Publishing Inc., Minneapolis, MN., ISBN: 978-1-57542-176-6, Page count: 40, Price: about $10. https://www.freespirit.com/early-childhood/talk-and-work-it-out-learning-to-get-along-cheri-meiners/

Lesson 15: Healthy choices

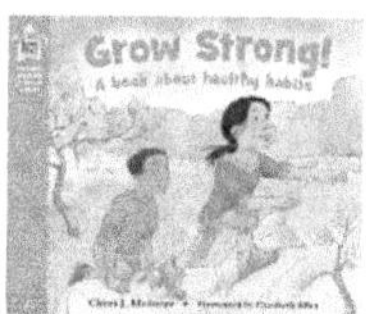

"Grow Strong!: A book about healthy habits" by Cheri J. Meiners, M.Ed. / illustrated by Elizabeth Allen, Free Spirit Publishing Inc., Minneapolis, MN. ISBN: 978-1-63198-085-5, Page count: 40, Price: about $10. https://www.freespirit.com/early-childhood/grow-strong-being-the-best-me-cheri-meiners-elizabeth-allen

EPILOGUE

"Cogito, ergo sum" (*"I think, therefore I am"*) is a philosophical proposition by René Descartes in the mid-17th century. Descartes' view became the foundation of contemporary philosophy, including the mind-body dualism which draws a clear distinction between mind and body. According to this view, the body cannot think and the mind can exist outside of the body. This idea leads to the notion of mental health as an illness of mind, which helped creating mental health stigma in the past. Today, recent advances in neuroscience finally allow us to think of mental health as a biochemical condition of the brain, not an illness of the mind.

Still, we are struggling with handling of mental health in large population. Perhaps, one way to eliminate stigma and clear our path toward better social emotional well-being is to think *"I feel, therefore I am."* The current mental healthcare focuses on suppressing symptoms, as if all bad feelings are to be eliminated. Instead, if we acknowledge that all feelings are natural and acceptable, perhaps we can shift our focus from symptoms to risk and protective factors as a balance regulator. This systems view may open a door to new opportunities and better solutions. Mental health is the most stigmatized topic in healthcare, and I hope that the book brought clarity, structure, and positive outlook.

Sometimes too many words can dilute an important message: *you're not alone and there is hope.* Hope is the best positive influencer of all time. Thank you for reading.

Satoru Isaka

San Jose, California

June 2018

ABOUT THE AUTHOR

Satoru Isaka is a systems scientist and techno-philanthropist. Satoru received his Ph.D. in Systems Science from the University of California, San Diego. He was an active youth sports coach in baseball, softball, and soccer while raising his three children; he has the first-hand experience in the "filling the emotional tank" concept by Positive Coaching Alliance. With over 30 years of experience in research and development, he is applying his skills and knowledge in systems science to build technical solutions for public benefits.

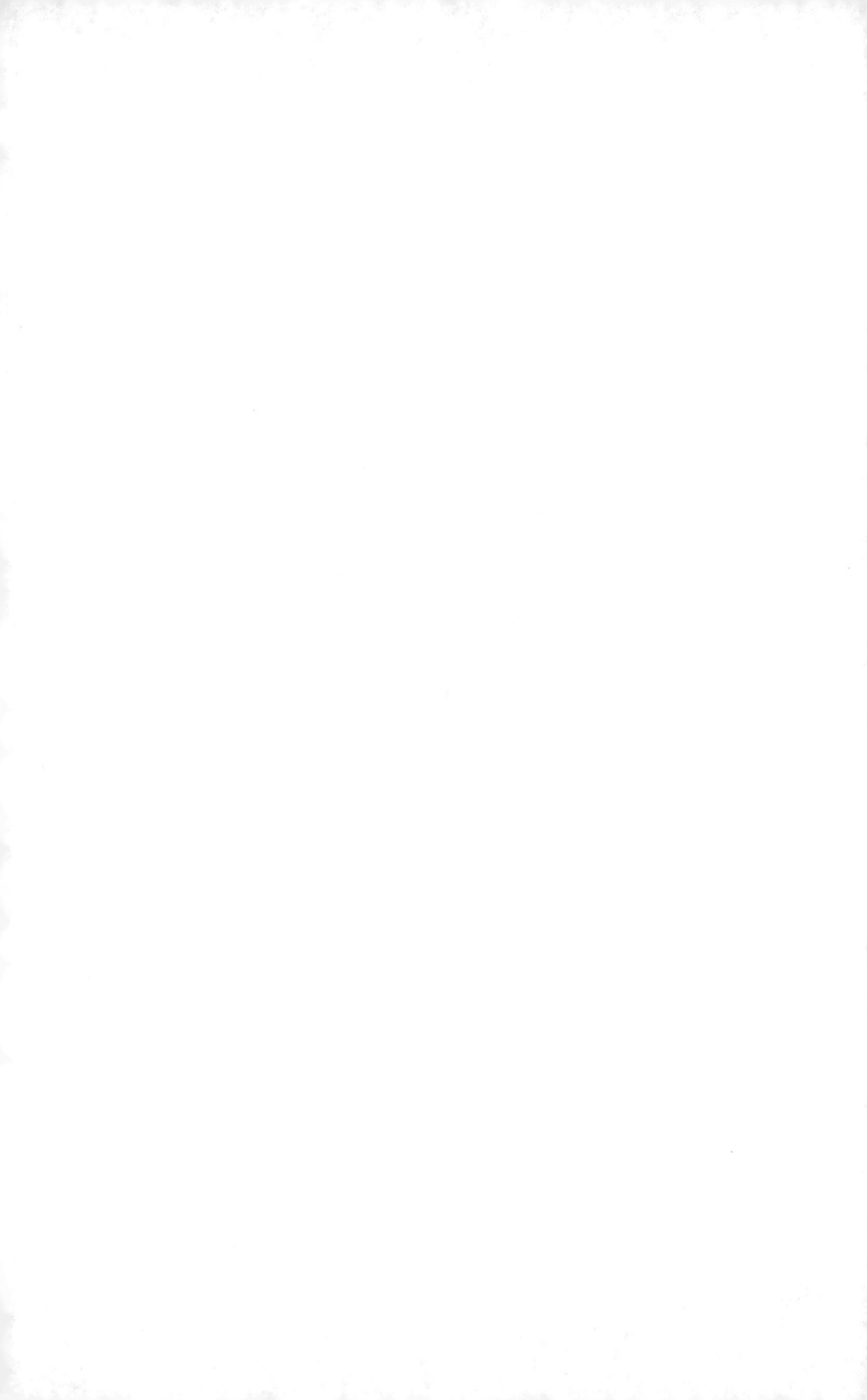

www.ingramcontent.com/pod-product-compliance
Lightning Source LLC
Chambersburg PA
CBHW060053260726
48658CB00004B/1282